CP"Teach"

Textbook

WRITTEN BY:

Patrice Morin-Spatz

Updated and Published Annually!

MedBooks
101 West Buckingham Road
Richardson, Texas 75081
1-800-443-7397
972-643-1809

www.medbooks.com

PREFACE

CP"Teach" was written with one single objective: to teach coders how to properly code "according to the book" (the **CPT** manual).

It is our experience, in years of dealing with thousands of coders nationwide, that proper coding results in many benefits to the physician's office. Among them are optimum reimbursement, which increases revenues, the recovery of "lost" (previously un-billed) dollars, and increased staff efficiency because coding properly decreases time spent dealing with reimbursables and claim filing.

For best results, we recommend that you follow each chapter along with the current edition of the **CPT** manual at your fingertips. This will allow you to learn by doing. Look up the examples given in **CP"Teach"** in the **CPT** manual and digest them before moving on to the next example.

ACKNOWLEDGEMENTS

Bill Kantz

CP"Teach" has been illustrated by talented artist Bill Kantz. Mr. Kantz's approach to his life's work was that "it's only worth doing if it's fun," and so we were excited that he opted to illustrate our book. Watercolor and pen & ink were among his favorite art mediums. Mr. Kantz provided illustrations on a national scale for several major firms including major oil & gas companies, Coca-Cola Foods, and Post and Kellogg's cereals. Mr. Kantz passed away in January of 2001 from cancer. His wit, style and playful nature will be greatly missed.

<u>DEDICATED TO</u>:

Calla

<u>DEDICATION</u>

This year, **CP"Teach"** is dedicated to wisdom. Dedicated to that because in it one has the keys to growth, maturity, and the ability to give up on old things while reaching for the new ones. Wisdom inspires anyone at the crossroads of life to reach for those opportunities that are so very scary but at the same time beckon for you to take hold of them. Wisdom is the calling of God, the listening to ones own internal power; it is the true core of us all.

Last year, I stood at the crossroads of my life. Afraid to face the future and afraid to let go of the past. Life gives us our twists and not always in the way we want them but always in the way we need them. I learned that when I asked for strength so that I might achieve, I was made weak so that I may learn to humbly obey. When I asked for help that I might do greater things, I was given humility to appreciate the work of others. When I asked for riches that I might be happy, I was given reality that I might be wise. When I asked for power and acknowledgement that I might have the praise of others, I was given weakness that I might know the need for God. I asked for all things that I might enjoy life and I was given life to enjoy all things. I have gotten little that I have asked for but everything that I hoped for and even despite myself, my deepest prayers have been answered.

OTHER MEDBOOKS PRODUCTS

CP"Teach" Student Textbook ISBN0-923369-76-7
Updated Each Year! $47.95

This is an excellent teaching tool for use both in the classroom and on an individual basis. Not only can it be used to learn **CPT** from the beginning, but it can also be used to brush up on skills for the experienced coder. Used by over 900 colleges, universities and technical schools as their text for teaching **CPT**.

CP"Teach" Workbook ISBN0-923369-77-5
Updated Each Year! $32.95

A self-motivated person could become an expert **CPT** coder by using **CP"Teach"** and the **CP"Teach"** Workbook. Filled with fun yet challenging exercises, this workbook will provide the user with in-depth study of **CPT** coding principles.

CP"Teach" Workbook with Answers ISBN0-923369-78-3
Updated Each Year! $39.95

CP"Teach" Instructor's Manual & Mylar Transparencies ISBN0-923369-79-1
$199.95
Updated Each Year!

Written for the manager or college instructor who is required to teach **CPT** coding, the manual contains course outlines, overhead transparencies, homework assignments, chapter quizzes and a final exam complete with answer guides. It is now being used in more than 500 colleges and universities to train medical assistants, insurance personnel and health information management professionals.

CP"Teach" Instructor's Manual & Paper Patterns to Make Transparencies ISBN0-923369-80-5
$149.95
Updated Each Year!

Case Study Workbook ISBN0-923369-57-0
$39.95

The **Case Study Workbook** contains actual patient charts (some even with the doctor's handwriting) from a variety of specialties. The student is challenged to code each exercise as if he or she were working in the physician's office.

Case Study Workbook with Answers ISBN0-923369-58-9
$44.95

DISCLAIMER

Because each insurance company has its own processing and reimbursing policies, it is important to note that the thoughts and recommendations given in this book may not apply to each individual carrier. It is critical that you check with each of your carriers to determine the applicability of the ideas outlined herein and determine which practices are unique to that carrier and which may not follow the guidelines set forth in **CP"Teach"**.

CP"Teach"

Printed in the U.S.A.

ISBN: 0-923369-76-7

TABLE OF CONTENTS

CHAPTER ONE:
CPT Basics 1

CHAPTER TWO:
What is HCPCS? 7

CHAPTER THREE:
HCPCS: Editorial Notations 27

CHAPTER FOUR:
CPT: Format of the Book 51

CHAPTER FIVE:
CPT: Editorial Notations 73

CHAPTER SIX:
Evaluation and Management 95

CHAPTER SEVEN:
Surgery 207

CHAPTER EIGHT:
Radiology 319

CHAPTER NINE:
Pathology and Laboratory 339

CHAPTER TEN:
Medicine 363

CHAPTER ELEVEN:
Modifiers 411

CHAPTER TWELVE:
Completing the HCFA 1500 Claim Form for Medicare 461

INDEX: 499

CPT CODES

The **CP"Teach"** series includes some of the American Medical Association's **Physician's Current Procedural Terminology** descriptive terms, numeric identifying codes, and modifiers for reporting medical services and procedures that were identified by the author, MedBooks, for inclusion in this book. **Physician's Current Procedural Terminology** is copyrighted (1966, 1970, 1973, 1977, 1981, 1983, 1984, 1985, 1986, 1987, 1988, 1989, 1990, 1991, 1992, 1993, 1994, 1995, 1996, 1997, 1998, 1999, 2000, 2001, 2002) by the American Medical Association. Any use of the **CPT** outside **CP"Teach"** should refer to **CPT** as it contains the most current listings of the descriptive terms, numeric services, and procedures.

Suggestions on code additions or deletions in **CPT** should be directed to the American Medical Association at the following address:

Information and Education Services
CPT
American Medical Association
515 North State Street
Chicago, Illinois 60610
800-634-6922
312-464-5022

DISCLAIMER

Because each insurance company has its own processing and reimbursing policies, it is important to note that the thoughts and recommendations given in this book may not apply to each individual carrier. It is critical that you check with each of your carriers to determine the applicability of the ideas outlined herein and determine which practices are unique to that carrier and which may not follow the guidelines set forth in **CP"Teach"**.

CHAPTER ONE

CPT BASICS

CPT, or *Current Procedural Terminology*, is a book used to code the procedures and services performed by physicians. It contains a listing of all current and FDA (Food and Drug Administration) approved physician procedures and services. Individual *code numbers* have been assigned to identify all procedures and services.

Here is an example of a **CPT** code and its corresponding service:

99201 *Office and other outpatient visit for the evaluation and management of a new patient, which requires these three key components:*

- *a problem-focused history;*
- *a problem-focused exam; and*
- *straightforward medical decision-making.*

> *Counseling and/or coordination of care with other providers or agencies are provided consistent with the nature of the problem(s) and the patient's and/or family's needs.*
>
> *Usually, the presenting problem(s) are self-limited or minor. Physicians typically spend 10 minutes face-to-face with the patient and/or family.*
>
> Copyright AMA, 2002

As you can see, the number 99201 identifies a specific service, in this case for a new patient. The service identified in the code 99201 is the history and exam that includes focusing on one, and only one, patient problem. Examples of a singular problem (in which a physician can make a straightforward decision and is not necessarily concerned with other patient problems) may include a history and exam for keratosis of the upper back or a patient who has an impacted wisdom tooth. No other procedure or service has this particular number. That is, the code 99201 will always mean, to the computer and to the coder, a problem-focused history and exam with straightforward decision-making for a new patient office or outpatient visit.

A different code is assigned to every service and every procedure that a physician performs. In this way, each procedure or service can be identified by a number instead of a lengthy written description.

The **CPT** book was born as a result of conversations between the American Medical Association and various other organiza-

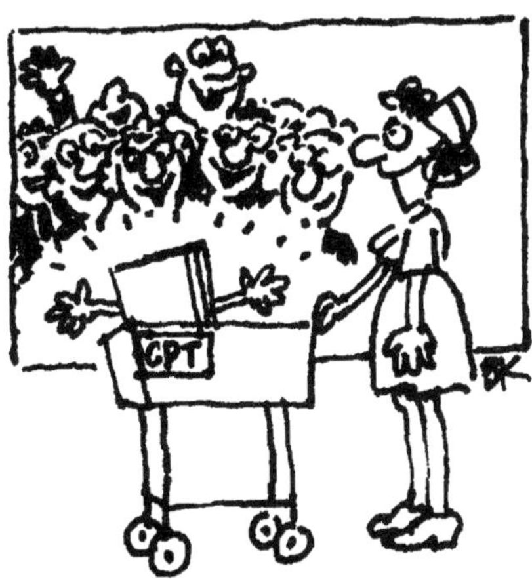

*The **CPT** book was born as a result of conversations between the American Medical Association and various other organizations.*

tions, such as the Executive Committee of the National Association of Blue Shield Plans; the Committee on Fees of the California Medical Association; the College of American Pathologists; the American College of Radiology; the American Society of Internal Medicine; the Health Insurance Council and the U.S. Department of Health, Education, and Welfare. All of these groups were interested in simplifying the reporting of diagnostic and therapeutic procedures provided by physicians to patients. More effectively, they wanted a way in which they could understand what procedures the doctor had provided to the patient without having to read a lengthy report.

By having a code for each individual procedure provided by the doctor to the patient, insurance carriers across the country would be able to do several things, including:

1. Communicate more effectively with each other;
2. Compare reimbursable amounts for procedures;
3. Speed the processing of claims.

Because the codes on the claims would be read, interpreted, and reimbursed by computer rather than by people (e.g., individual data processors, although the data processors would in many cases input the data), these carriers would be able to reduce the manpower needed for claims processing.

Throughout the 1960s and 1970s, the popularity of **CPT** as a coding tool was limited. It wasn't until the early 1980s that the **CPT** book really came into its own when Congress decided to use **CPT** for the coding of all physician procedures and services provided to Medicare patients.

Although **CPT** described physician procedures and services, it did not include some other items which needed to be reported to Medicare such as ambulance service, wheelchairs, and an extensive list of drugs used for individual injections. Because of **CPT**'s limitations, the Health Care Financing Administration (HCFA) at that time invented a common coding system. HCFA ran the Medicare program under the federal government's Department of Health, Education, and Welfare, now called the Department of Health and Human Services. HCFA changed its name on June 14, 2001 and is now called CMS or Centers for Medicare and Medicaid Services. The HCPCS coding system would employ **CPT** for the coding of physicians' procedures and services, but second and third levels would be added to provide a method of coding items *not* found in **CPT**.

This common coding system was called HCPCS pronounced "HICPICS". It stands for the following:

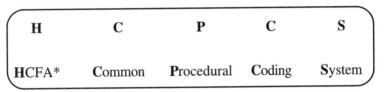

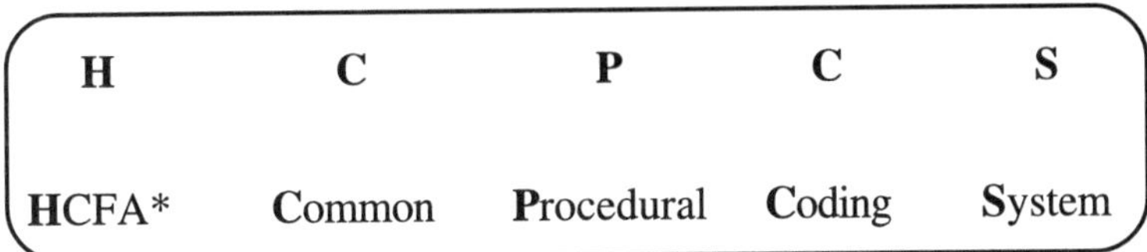
H C P C S
HCFA* Common Procedural Coding System

*HCFA = Health Care Financing Administration, now called CMS = Centers for Medicare and Medicaid Services.

CPT is updated annually because medicine is changing rapidly, new procedures are made available, older ones are being used less frequently, and other procedures need to be more accurately described. By updating the **CPT** manual each year, the AMA is able to make the appropriate changes they feel best represent today's medical practice. This flexibility has proved beneficial.

Coders often wonder if they should spend the money each year to purchase a new volume of **CPT**. Because of the annual changes, the current year's volume of **CPT** is a *critical* addition to your office library. Without the current book, your office runs the risk of missing one of the changes, which places your reimbursements at risk.

CHAPTER TWO

WHAT IS HCPCS?

HCPCS is an acronym that stands for **HCFA Common Procedural Coding System**.

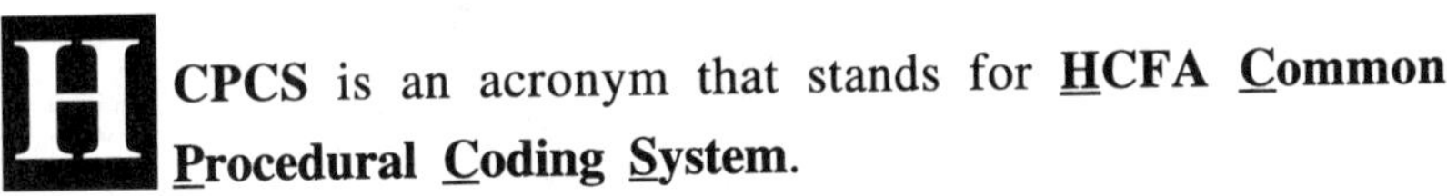

H C P C S
HCFA Common Procedural Coding System

HCFA itself is an acronym that represents the Center for Medicare and Medicaid Services, CMS, formerly known as Health Care Financing Administration. Most people pronounce the acronym 'HICFA"rather than saying each letter. This agency administers the Medicare, Medicaid and State Children's Health Insurance Program (SCHIP) as well as the

Health Insurance Portability and Accountability Act (HIPAA) programs. For more information about CMS, see **http://cms.hhs.gov**.

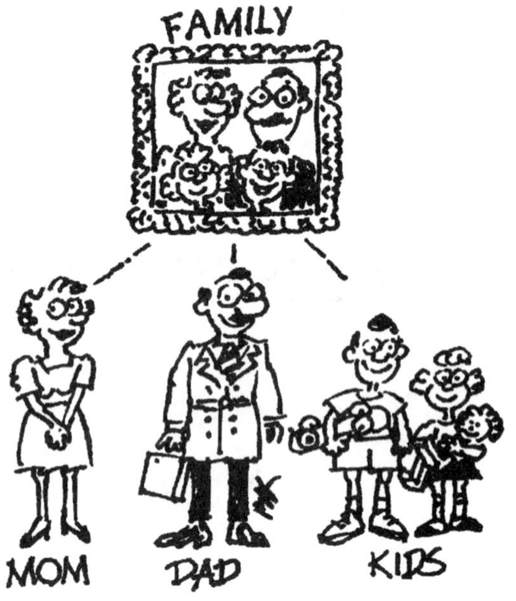

HCPCS, like a family, is really three different groups in one global system.

HCPCS describes members of one system. The current members of the HCPCS family are **CPT** Codes, National Codes, and Local Codes.

CPT Codes are also considered to be Level I of HCPCS. They are published yearly by the American Medical Association and are used for billing procedures and services performed by physicians. Since the federal government did not want to reinvent the wheel, it adopted **CPT** as the standard for coding procedures.

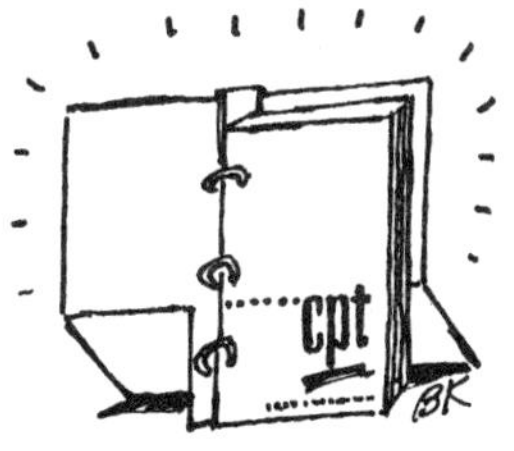

National Codes are the Level II of HCPCS. They are published yearly by the Medicare program in a book called the **National Coding Manual**. There are many vendors who produce the **National Coding Manual** (AKA HCPCS). Make sure you get one that gives you the payment information you need (usually found in the right hand column of the book). National Codes are used to bill for procedures and services that include dental work, durable medical equipment, injections, ophthalmological services, orthotics, some pathology and laboratory services, some rehabilitation services, many supplies, and vision care. Remember, National Codes were invented to provide CMS with a way of billing procedures and supplies for Medicare patients. Because many private carriers run the Medicare program for CMS and also administer their own programs to their own patients, they most likely use the National Codes.

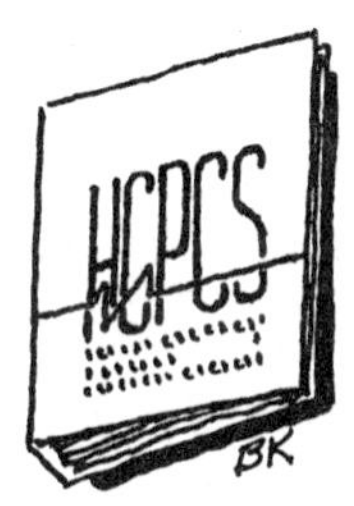

Local Codes are also called Level III codes. These codes and descriptions describe procedures and services that usually do not exist in **CPT** or the **National Coding Manual**. Local Codes could also describe procedures and services coded by Medicare, which the carriers feel are better described through the use of another code. Local Codes are developed on an as-needed basis (rather than once a year) by the local (statewide) Medicare carrier and replace unlisted procedure codes, which cost carriers excessive time and energy to process. Local codes must be approved by CMS before being implemented.

To place the three components of the HCPCS coding system into perspective, it is important to compare and contrast them in order to see where the coding systems are alike and where they differ.

Take a look at the table on the next page. If a procedure, service, or supply is coded extensively enough for the Medicare program by a **CPT** code, an “X” appears under the heading "Found in **CPT**" in the table. If it is better described elsewhere, an “X” appears under the second heading, “Better Found Elsewhere.”

In reviewing this list, you can see that many services and supplies your physician may provide are not extensively coded for in **CPT**. For example, supplies like surgical trays or fiberglass for casting are not readily identified using a **CPT** code. Because of this, it is important to understand the entire range of HCPCS coding and to realize that **CPT** is only a part of this system.

To give you clearer insight into the HCPCS coding system, let’s further examine the three levels of codes that make up this system.

Procedures and Services Coded by Medicare		
	Found in **CPT**	Better Found Elsewhere
Ambulance Services		X
Chiropractic	X	X
Chemotherapeutic Drugs		X
Consultations	X	
Dental	X	X
Durable Medical Equipment		X
Hospital Visits	X	
Injections (Drugs)	X	X
Office Visits	X	
Opthalmological Services	X	X
Orthotics/Prosthetics		X
Pathology/Laboratory	X	
Rehabilitation Services	X	X
Supplies		X
Surgery	X	
Vision Services	X	X

How CPT is Divided

The **CPT** book is divided into seven major sections that appear in the following order: Evaluation and Management, Anesthesia, Surgery, Radiology, Pathology and Laboratory, and Medicine. There are other major sections that appear in **CPT** (e.g., the appendices) that we will not talk about here. There is no apparent reason for this particular order, but an easy way to memorize it is to consider the steps involved in the medical treatment process:

1. First, the patient comes to the office to find out what the problem is (Evaluation and Management Section).

2. Once it is decided that the patient needs an operation, he or she is anesthetized (Anesthesia Section).

3. After the patient is "under," the surgery begins (Surgery Section).

4. The patient might be undergoing a diagnostic surgical procedure that requires intervention and assistance of a radiologist (Radiology Section).

5. The patient might be undergoing a biopsy which requires the assistance of a pathologist. Upon its removal from the patient, the specimen is taken to the laboratory for examination (Pathology and Laboratory Section).

6. Often, the patient is released from the hospital with prescriptions for several kinds of nonsurgical treatments or tests, such as EKGs, psychological testing, or physical therapy (Medicine Section).*

7. Category III codes take into account procedures that may be in the developmental or experimental phases. These codes begin with the number 00 and usually end with the letter T (temporary). Their placement in the book may be for a year, or more or they may be incorporated into the regular text of the **CPT** book as the procedure they represent becomes less "temporary" and more universally used in the practice of medicine.

*Prior to 1992, the Medicine Section was located at the beginning of the **CPT** book. In 1992, it was moved to the end of the book.

The different sections of **CPT** will be discussed in greater detail in later chapters of **CP"Teach"**.

The Logic of CPT Codes

All **CPT** codes are composed of five numeric digits (numbers). The first number in a **CPT** code depends on the section in which the code is found.

- Codes in the **Evaluation and Management Section** begin with **9**.
- Codes in the **Anesthesia Section** begin with **0**.

- Codes in the **Surgery Section** begin with **1**, **2**, **3**, **4**, **5**, and **6**.
- Codes in the **Radiology Section** begin with **7**.
- Codes in the **Pathology and Laboratory Section** begin with **8**.
- Codes in the **Medicine Section** begin with **9**.
- Category three codes begin with the number 00 and end with the letter T.

As you can see, except for Evaluation and Management, the first digits of the codes in the sections are in numerical order. Anesthesia codes begin with the number 0; Surgery codes begin with numbers from 1 through 6, etc.

Examples of CPT Codes

The number **9**, the first digit of all codes in the Evaluation and Management Section and the Medicine Section, identifies a noninvasive procedure or service. Following is an example of an Evaluation and Management code:

99291 *Critical care, evaluation and management of the critically ill or critically injured patient; first 30 - 74 minutes*

The first digit of a code in the Anesthesia Section is "0". An example of an Anesthesia code is:

00100 Anesthesia for procedures on salivary glands, including biopsy

Qualifying circumstance codes for anesthesia can be found both in the Anesthesia and Medicine Sections of the **CPT** book. These are important in billing for an anesthesiologist since they help clarify the patient's condition (e.g., anesthesia for patient of extreme age). These codes range from number 99100 through number 99140. Other codes that have to do with sedation (99141 and 99142) are also found in the Medicine Section and not in the Anethesia Section.

The fact that codes in the Surgery Section begin with the numbers **1**, **2**, **3**, **4**, **5**, and **6** may seem unimportant. However, each section of **CPT** has its own set of rules. Within the Surgery Section, each beginning number says something about the type of procedure being coded. Knowing the first digit of a code will give you a clue about the rules required to bill the procedure or service properly.

Examples of Surgery codes include:

10140 Incision and drainage of hematoma; seroma or fluid collection*

20200 Biopsy, muscle; superficial

30115 Excision, nasal polyp(s), extensive

40840 *Vestibuloplasty; anterior*

50045 *Nephrotomy, with exploration*

61304 *Craniectomy or craniotomy, exploratory; supratentorial*

As you can see, procedures described in this section are basically invasive procedures. It is in the Surgery Section that you will find incisions, excisions, repairs, biopsies, punctures, aspirations, explorations, destructions, introductions, and removals.

The Radiology Section begins with the number "**7**" and includes Diagnostic Radiology (Diagnostic Imaging), Diagnostic Ultrasound, Radiation Oncology, and Nuclear Medicine.

Following is an example of a Radiology code:

70490 *Computerized tomography, soft tissue neck; without contrast material*

The Pathology and Laboratory Section includes several subsections, including Automated Multichannel Tests, Chemistry and Toxicology, Hematology and Coagulation, and Immunology, just to name a few.

Following are examples of Pathology and Laboratory codes:

82308 *Calcitonin*

85097 *Bone marrow; smear interpretation*

Procedures and services found in the Medicine Section are generally noninvasive. That is, the codes describe cardiopulmonary resuscitation (CPR), allergy testing, psychiatric services, biofeedback, ophthalmology services and supplies, and a host of other procedures and services that generally don't involve cutting the patient or taking anything out.

Following is an example of a Medicine code:

92015 Determination of refractive state

Category III Codes

Following the Pathology Section are the Category III codes. These codes provide the user with an actual specific code to use for services that have not been adopted in the regular "text" portion of **CPT**. The services described by Category III codes are emerging services (new technologies or procedures that aren't yet widely used). These Category III codes are temporary codes and allow both the American Medical Association and Insurance Carriers to collect data on the usage of such procedures and services. If you are providing a service described by a Category III code, you should use it as opposed to an Unlisted Procedure Code. More information on Category III codes will be given later in Chapter Four, Format of the Book.

National Codes

Because **CPT** describes only physician procedures and services, CMS needed another method to code for supplies, injections, and other procedures and services it recognizes (but does not necessarily pay for) that were either not found in **CPT** or were not extensively coded. This is how National Codes came into being. CMS, with the help of the Health Insurance Association of America, Blue Cross Blue Shield and the American Dental Association who helped with the "D" codes (5 digit codes that start off with the letter "D" and describe dental services) took responsibility for deciding what codes and descriptions to place in the **National Coding Manual**.

How the National Coding Manual is Divided

Like **CPT,** the **National Coding Manual** is divided into sections. However, the sections are not like those in **CPT**. That is, they don't include Evaluation and Management, Anesthesia, etc. Instead, they cover such categories as Ambulance Services, Dental Procedures, Injections, Vision Services, and many others.

The Logic of National Codes

Like **CPT** codes, National Codes are composed of five digits. Unlike **CPT** codes, however, National Codes are alphanumeric. An alphanumeric code combines letters of the alphabet with numbers. In the case of National Codes, one letter is followed by four numbers.

Following is an example of a National Code:

A4550 Surgical tray

Just as the first digit of a **CPT** code is always a number from 0 through 9, the first digit of a National Code is always a letter from A through V.

Because there are so many sections of the **National Coding Manual**, the code numbers are split more generally than those of **CPT**. For example, codes starting with the letter "A" describe "**A**mbulance" Services and General Supplies; codes beginning with the letter "D," as mentioned earlier, refer to "**D**ental" Services; and codes starting with the letter "J" describe "In**J**ections."

Other codes are described in the **National Coding Manual**.

LOCAL CODES

As we said earlier, Local Codes were invented so that individual carriers could report, via codes, the development of trends in a particular state. For example, technological breakthroughs often lead to the use of procedures and services for which there are no codes in either **CPT** or the **National Coding Manual.**

Carriers needed the flexibility to invent codes for such procedures and services and Local Codes gave them that flexibility.

Local Codes must be approved for use by the Center for Medicare and Medicaid Services before being used on a local or statewide scale. CMS requires the authorization of Local Codes in order to better implement the OBRA law to make all coding and payment uniform. The government feels that this movement toward a uniform coding system and payment policy will ensure that all coding among all physicians in all states is consistent. This will aid CMS in reporting to taxpayers all costs associated with all governmentally insured programs.

Currently, the letters W, X, Y, and Z are reserved for Local Codes.

To place the different parts of the HCPCS coding system into perspective, let's look at the following table. We will be able to see at a glance how they are alike and how they differ.

H C P C S		
CPT **Level I**	**NATIONAL** **Level II**	**LOCAL** **Level III**
Developed by AMA	Developed by CMS, formerly known as HCFA	Developed by state carriers
Divided into 7 sections	Divided into 17 sections	Not divided
Sections include:	Sections include:	
Evaluation and Management Anesthesia Surgery Radiology Pathology/Lab Medicine Category III	Ambulance Services Chiropractic Supplies Miscellaneous Dental Durable Medical Home Health Rehabilitation Injections Chemotherapeutic Drugs Orthotics/Prosthetics Medical Pathology/Lab Radiology Surgery Vision Hearing	
5-digit numeric with the exception of Category III codes that end in a letter	5-digit alphanumeric; codes begin with a letter	5-digit alphanumeric
e.g., 99201	e.g., A4550	e.g., W1000
first digit = 0-9	first digit = A-V	first digit = W-Z
describes physician procedures/services	describes physician procedures/services/ supplies/injections	describes physician procedures/services/ supplies
Updated annually	Updated annually	Updated as needed Approved by CMS
Printed annually	Printed annually	Printed as needed Found in bulletins released by Medicare carriers

Summary

CHAPTER TWO

✓ HCPCS is a system used by Medicare for the coding of procedures, services, and supplies for Medicare patients.

✓ HCPCS is composed of three separate coding systems. These include **CPT** codes (Level I), National Codes (Level II), and Local Codes (Level III).

✓ CMS must approve the assignment of any Local Codes.

✓ **CPT** codes are five-digit numeric codes beginning with the numbers 0 through 9. The sections in **CPT** have the following coding structure:

Section	**First Digit**
Evaluation and Management	9
Anesthesia	0
Surgery	1 through 6
Radiology	7
Pathology and Laboratory	8
Medicine	9

- ✓ National Codes are five-digit alphanumeric codes beginning with the letters A through V.

- ✓ Local Codes are five-digit alphanumeric codes beginning with the letters W through Z.

- ✓ **CPT** best describes physicians' procedures and services. It is updated once a year and usually becomes available in November/December of the preceding year.

- ✓ National Codes describe physicians' procedures as well as supplies, materials, and drugs for injections. These codes are found in the **HCPCS National Coding Manual**, which is usually made available by various vendors at approximately the same time as the **CPT** book.

- ✓ Local Codes are established and assigned on an as-needed basis. They are published by carriers in the bulletins they send to physicians and suppliers.

- ✓ Category III codes are temporary codes that should be used in place of unlisted procedures codes (if possible).

✓ Category III codes start off with a number (like all **CPT** codes) but end with the letter "T" which indicates that they are "temporary" codes and may not be around in future years. Permanent codes may be assigned to describe this service and replace the Category III code.

CHAPTER THREE

HCPCS: EDITORIAL NOTATIONS

Note: The examples used in this section were taken from the 2003 official Medicare version of the ***HCPCS National Coding Manual.***

The purpose of this chapter is to explain some of the peculiari- found in the **HCPCS National Coding Manual**. If you don't already have a copy, you must obtain one as soon as possible. The official Medicare version of the **HCPCS National Coding Manual** is available from both MedBooks (in CD form with the ability to print it yourself or in paper form) and from U.S. Government Printing Office.

HCPCS National Codes are five-digit, alphanumeric codes (e.g., A4550) used mainly for the coding of supplies, prosthetics, and drugs usually *not* found in **CPT**.

The **HCPCS National Coding Manual** is not hard to use. As we already discussed, the proper use of the **HCPCS National Coding Manual** is critical for full and accurate coding.

There are many fields (or explanations/further information given) that Medicare has made available to you in this book. See example below.

HCPC	Long Description	Action Code	Coverage Field	Statute	X-Ref	PI	ASC Pay Grp
A0021	AMBULANCE SERVICE, OUTSIDE STATE PER MILE, TRANSPORT (MEDICAID ONLY)	N	I		A0030	00	
A0030	AMBULANCE SERVICE, CONVENTIONAL AIR SERVICE, TRANSPORT, ONE WAY	N	I		A0430	00	
A0040	AMBULANCE SERVICE, AIR, HELICOPTER SERVICE, TRANSPORT	N	I		A0431	00	
A0050	AMBULANCE SERVICE, EMERGENCY, WATER, SPECIAL TRANSPORTATION SERVICES	N	I		A0429	00	

Most of these fields in the regular Medicare version of the HCPCS National Codes do not have any application for the regular coder who codes on a daily basis. In the CD Rom published by MedBooks (see **www.MedBooks.com**, or call 1-800-443-7397), we have taken away most of the "fluff" (removing fields that will have nothing to do with your coding) and given you the information that you need to make coding selections as easy and effective as possible and those that give you the needed information to complete the HCFA 1500 claim form or the UB 92. That being said, there are several "fields" that you need to be made aware of. These include the following (in the order in which they appear on our CD):

1. **The HCPCS Field** This is the area where you will find a particular alpha-numeric code *or* a **HCPCS National Coding Manual** modifier. "HCPC" is an acronym (a word made out of the first letters of other words) that stands for ***H***eath Care Financing Administration (now known as CMS or Centers for Medicare and Medicaid Services) ***C***ommon ***P***rocedural ***C***ode. You will see that the codes here mostly describe supplies used by medical providers (e.g., durable medical equipment, drugs for injections, surgical trays) but they also can *and do* describe some procedures or services (e.g., venipuncture).

2. **Action Code Field** You can see that this field actually uses the words "Action Code" to describe itself. It is here that Medicare tells you what they have done (if anything) to the code. More information about the Action Code field will be discussed later in this chapter.

3. **Coverage Field** This field is denoted by the abbreviation COV. It basically describes whether or not a code is "covered" by Medicare. More information about this field will be discussed later in this chapter.

4. **Statute Field** This field tells you whether or not a procedure, service or supply is covered by Medicare statute. More information about this field will be discussed later in this chapter.

5. **X-Ref** This field stands for the cross-reference field. It is here that you will find out if there is another code that the one you are looking at can be cross-referenced to. This field will be important to you if you are looking at a newer version of the **HCPCS National Coding Manual** and comparing it to an older one where there may have been some deletion of codes which could be cross-referenced to new or different codes.

6. **PI** This acronym stands for the ***P***ricing ***I***ndicator field. It is here that Medicare tells you what methodology they used to come up with the price for the service, supply or procedure for the Part B portion of the Medicare program.

7. **ASC Payment Group** If you are using the **HCPCS National Coding Manual** for coding things in an ASC (ambulatory surgical center), this field will tell you what payment group the code falls into. Payment groups help determine the amount of reimbursement you will get for the code.

We will study each of these fields individually.

THE HCPCS FIELD

As was stated earlier, this field shows the coder what the code number is for the description they have selected. Consider the following example.

HCPC	Long Description	Action Code	Coverage Field	Statute	X-Ref	PI	ASC Pay Grp
A4550	SURGICAL TRAYS	N	D			11	

As you can see by looking under the HCPC field there is a code in our example, the code A4550. As you learn more about the **HCPCS National Coding Manual** you will note that the codes come in both alpha sequence (i.e., they start off with the letter A, then B, and so on) and then they come in numerical sequence (e.g., the A4550 comes before the code A4554).

ACTION CODE FIELD

The Action Code Field describes what has happened to the code. In other words, the code may have been added, discontinued, re-activated, etc. Each of the possibilities for what you may see in this field are described on the next page.

ACTION CODE FIELDS

A = Procedure or modifier ADDED to the text
B = Change in BOTH the administrative data field or in the long description of the procedure has been made
C = CHANGE in the long description of the procedure or modifier
D = The procedure or modifier code has been DISCONTINUED
F = There has been a change in *only* the administrative data FIELD
N = NO maintenance for this code
P = PAYMENT change
R = A discontinued or deleted procedure has been RE-ACTIVATED
S = There has been a change in the SHORT description version of the descriptions of the codes
T = Miscellaneous TYPE of change

Make sure that you read and understand each one of these notations as they can be important in your code selection. For example, suppose you went to select a code for a patient of yours who was incontinent. You had been using the code A4360 that stood for the following:

A4360 Adult incontinence garment (e.g., brief, diaper, etc.)

If you were to look at the following section from the **HCPCS National Coding Manual** you would see that the coverage field denotes that this supply code has been discontinued.

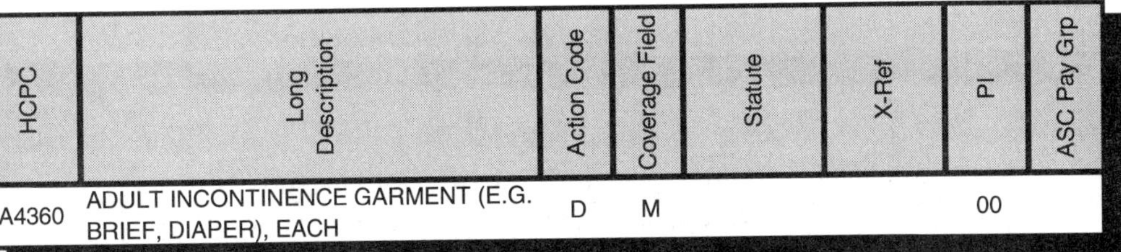

HCPC	Long Description	Action Code	Coverage Field	Statute	X-Ref	PI	ASC Pay Grp
A4360	ADULT INCONTINENCE GARMENT (E.G. BRIEF, DIAPER), EACH	D	M			00	

Seeing that the coverage of the code for this supply has been discontinued is important to you because it tells you that you should not use the code and, if had you previously been using the code, it alerts you to pick another code. Once a code is discontinued, you can use it all you want but the carrier will simply deny it.

As you will see in **CP 'Teach"** when we discuss the **CPT** editorial notations, there are some notations that bear special consideration. The notations in **HCPCS National Code Manual** include many of those listed above. For example, if you were to look at the A, (for the procedure or supply being "added"), you can easily see that the significance of a code with this notation would be great. In the first place, a code with an "A" lets you know that the code and its description are "new" to the book. Secondly, it tells you that the payment on the code will be newly established as well. Let's take an example.

HCPC	Long Description	Action Code	Coverage Field	Statute	X-Ref	PI	ASC Pay Grp
J3315	INJECTION, TRIPTORELIN PAMOATE, 3.75 MG	A	D			51	

As you can see by the example listed above, the coverage notation for J3315 shows an "A" in the field. This would be an example of a code that has been "added" for 2003.

Likewise, a code with a "C" on it will indicate that something about the description of the code has changed. A change in the description of the code could mean that the reimbursement amount may be different than it was in previous years. Be sure to look at all of the notations and when you review the **HCPCS National Coding Manual**, make sure that you look at the Coverage Field to see if any of notations apply to the code you are choosing. If there is a notation in the Coverage Field, make sure that you understand what it means and what its implications are for your reimbursement.

Keep in mind that what appears in the Coverage Field may not be as current as you suspect. Not all "A's" (for added codes) for instance have been added for the *current year*. Medicare does not always "clean out" the old and update all of the different fields. Keeping last year's version of the **HCPCS National Coding Manual** will help you sort out these issues for yourself and assist you in being able to tell what actions have been taken on the code for a particular year. If you are new to coding and do not have a library of former versions of both **CPT** and the **HCPCS National Coding Manuals**, start this year by beginning to keep one.

Coverage Field

This field will give you important information about the coverage of a particular code. There are several "coverage" notations that you will need to know. These can be found in the chart that follows.

Coverage Fields
C = Carrier judgment
D = Special coverage instructions apply
G = Not valid for Medicare (90-day grace period)
I = Not valid for Medicare (no grace period)
M = Non-covered by Medicare
S = Non-covered by Medicare Statute

If you really think about it, each of the initials for "coverage" implies something. For example, the "C" stands for ***C***arrier judgment, the "D" can almost be thought of as ***D***enial of the claim unless special circumstances apply (e.g., the service is a starred service or the supply is not normally part of the service), the "G" can be thought of as the fact the a ***G***race period applies and so on. These notations are very important to understand as the selection of the code in the **HCPCS National Coding Manual** will depend upon (in many cases) whether or not you will get paid for whatever you are coding. Let us take each of these individually and discuss their meaning.

C = CARRIER JUDGMENT

A service or supply with the "C" notation (Carrier Judgment) simply means that the Medicare carrier may *or may not* elect to pay for the service, supply or procedure to which it is attached. Many times, the decision to reimburse a claim with a code that has this notation on it is based upon what diagnosis code you submit on your claim. An example of the "C" notation is the following.

HCPC	Long Description	Action Code	Coverage Field	Statute	X-Ref	PI	ASC Pay Grp
AW	ITEM FURNISHED IN CONJUNCTION WITH A SURGICAL DRESSING	A	C				
AX	ITEM FURNISHED IN CONJUNCTION WITH DIALYSIS SERVICES	A	C				
BA	ITEM FURNISHED IN CONJUNCTION WITH PARENTERAL ENTERAL NUTRITION (PEN) SERVICES	A	C				

M = Not Covered by Medicare
S = Not Covered by Medicare Statute

If a service is non-covered by Medicare Statute (see notation "S"), it means that you cannot bill the patient for it at all. This is different from not being covered by Medicare (see notation "M"). When a supply, procedure or service is not covered by Medicare, it can be billed to the patient, it is just that Medicare will not pay for it. When you see that the supply, service or procedure that you want to code is not covered by "Medicare Statute" (see notation "S"), keep in mind that although you won't bill it for a Medicare patient, you may be allowed (by some carriers) to bill it for a non-Medicare patient.

HCPC	Long Description	Action Code	Coverage Field	Statute	X-Ref	PI	ASC Pay Grp
GX	SERVICE NOT COVERED BY MEDICARE	N	M				
GY	ITEM OR SERVICE STATUTORILY EXCLUDED OR DOES NOT MEET THE DEFINITION OF ANY 'MEDICARE BENEFIT	N	S				
GZ	ITEM OR SERVICE EXPECTED TO BE DENIED AS NOT REASONABLE AND NECESSARY	N	M				

G = Not Valid for Medicare (90-Day Grace Period)
I = Not Valid for Medicare (No Grace Period)

A code with the "G" in the Coverage field means that the Medicare carrier does not allow the code but that they are making it available to non-Medicare carriers and that they will allow you to use it for a period of 90 days from the effective change date. Use of the code after that time will not be allowed or, in the event that you do use it, the code will just be ignored by Medicare. Similarly, the "I" means the same thing in that should you use this code choice, Medicare will simply choose to "ignore" it. It bears repeating that just because Medicare will not recognize a code does not mean that you should not use it. There may be other carriers that recognize the code and even if they do not, the patient may be responsible for paying for the supply, procedure or service.

HCPC	Long Description	Action Code	Coverage Field	Statute	X-Ref	PI	ASC Pay Grp
A0021	AMBULANCE SERVICE, OUTSIDE STATE PER MILE, TRANSPORT (MEDICAID ONLY)	N	I		A0030	00	
A0030	AMBULANCE SERVICE, CONVENTIONAL AIR SERVICE, TRANSPORT, ONE WAY	N	I		A0430	00	
A0040	AMBULANCE SERVICE, AIR, HELICOPTER SERVICE, TRANSPORT	N	I		A0431	00	
A0050	AMBULANCE SERVICE, EMERGENCY, WATER, SPECIAL TRANSPORTATION SERVICES	N	I		A0429	00	

STATUTE FIELD

This is the field were you will find out where in the **Medicare Carrier's Manual** the rule is for services that are not covered by Medicare Statute or simply not covered by Medicare. Knowing the difference between these two (not covered by Medicare Statute and not covered by Medicare) is easy. All you have to know is that if a code is not covered by Medicare statute, you cannot:

1. Bill the supply or service to a Medicare patient;
2. Medicare will not *cover* the supply, procedure or service for the patient.

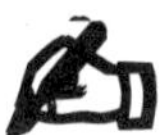

A procedure, supply or service that is not covered by Medicare Statute can only be billed to a non-Medicare patient.

This information will come from the **Medicare Carrier's Manual** which you should obtain if you are providing procedures, services or supplies for which there is a notation in this Medicare Statute Field that you feel is important. Otherwise, keep in mind that the likelihood that you will get any reimbursement from Medicare on these items is nil.

Cross Reference

You will see some examples of the Cross Reference codes (see X-Ref) below.

HCPC	Long Description	Action Code	Coverage Field	Statute	X-Ref	PI	ASC Pay Grp
A0021	AMBULANCE SERVICE, OUTSIDE STATE PER MILE, TRANSPORT (MEDICAID ONLY)	N	I		A0030	00	
A0030	AMBULANCE SERVICE, CONVENTIONAL AIR SERVICE, TRANSPORT, ONE WAY	N	I		A0430	00	
A0040	AMBULANCE SERVICE, AIR, HELICOPTER SERVICE, TRANSPORT	N	I		A0431	00	

As you can see by looking at these, the original HCPCS National Code is cross-referenced to another code that you can ***use in place of*** the one that is the actual HCPCS code you are looking at.

For example, if you look at the first code, A0021 for a per mile charge for transfer of a Medicaid patient via ambulance service outside the state, you will note that in the X-Ref field it says A0030. As you can see, this code, A0030 also has a cross-reference to another code, A0430. Seeing this will give you an example of what we spoke about earlier; that being that Medicare does not always update its own files. It would not make sense to most of us that the cross reference we would get would send us to something that is cross referenced yet again, however, in this example, this is the case.

Additionally, you can also see by looking at both the Action Code field and the Coverage field that both of these codes, A0021 and A0030, are not valid for Medicare (see COV = I) *and*, that Medicare is not responsible for maintaining these codes. (Both the COV and Action Code notations make sense when you look at the description of the code and realize that in at least one example the service was provided to a Medicaid (not Medicare) patient.)

Make sure that you continue to follow the X-Ref's and find out what the final stop is. For example, after you looked at the first code, A0021, you were cross-referenced to the second code, A0030 which then cross-referenced you to a third code, A0430. Continue on your search until you have un-earthed all of the cross-references possible. Also check the other fields to make sure that the code you finally come up with is valid for use and can be placed on your claim form.

Pricing Indicator

If you are curious about how Medicare came up with the fees for various supplies, procedures and services under Medicare Part B, the PI field will help you understand. In the field for PI you may find a two-digit code that will mean something to Medicare. You will see a complete list of all pricing indicators to follow.

You will note that the pricing indicators are two-digits (e.g., 11). An 11 in the field for PI would indicate to you (and to the carriers) that the pricing for this particular supply, procedure or service was made based on using the national relative value units. (Relative values to insurance companies are what "pounds" are to your local grocer. That is, if you know how many pounds something weighs, you can determine (if you have the price per pound) how much to charge (or what the cost is) for the meat (or vegetables) you want to buy.) Similarly, the relative values measure how much time, practice overhead, physician expertise, and malpractice costs are associated with codes. If you then know the "price per pound" (which may be different for office visits, versus surgeries versus supplies, etc), you can figure out how much the value of the overall code is by multiplying the relative value (number of pounds) by the value for that kind of supply, procedure or service. What is important for you to note right now is *not* how you calculate a relative value, but rather *that* it exists and is used to calculate fees.

There are twenty-five pricing indicators found in the **HCPCS National Coding Manual**. These are listed below. You will see that there are different groupings of pricing indicators which are important to pay attention to. For example, those PI which fall into the Clinical Lab Fee Schedule are unique to supplies, procedures and services for lab.

PRICING INDICATORS

00 Services are not covered, bundled or are used in Part A Medicare only and are not priced separately by Medicare Part B

LINKED TO PHYSICIAN FEE SCHEDULE

11 Price established using national relative value units

12 Price established using national anesthesia base units

13 Price established by carriers and at their discretion

CLINICAL LAB FEE SCHEDULE

21 Price subject to national limitation amount

22 Price established by carriers and at their discretion

SUPPLIES AND SURGICAL DRESSINGS

31 Frequently serviced durable medical equipment (DME) (price subject to floors and ceilings)

32 Inexpensive and routinely purchased DME (price subject to floors and ceilings)

33 Oxygen and oxygen equipment (price subject to floors and ceilings)

34 DME supplies (price subject to floors and ceilings)

35 Surgical dressings (price subject to floors and ceilings)

36	Capped rental DME (price subject to floors and ceilings)
37	Ostomy, tracheostomy and urological supplies (price subject to floors and ceilings)
38	Orthotics, prosthetics, prosthetic devices and vision services (price subject to floors and ceilings)
39	Parenteral and Enteral Nutrition
45	Customized DME items
46	Carrier priced

OTHER

51	Drugs
52	Reasonable charge
53	Statute
54	Vaccinations
55	Priced by carriers under clinical psychologist fee schedule (not applicable as of January 1998)
56	Priced by carriers under clinical social worker fee schedule (not applicable as of January 1998)
57	Other carrier priced
99	Value not established

If you check out the example below, you will see the PI field for the code C1012.

HCPC	Long Description	Action Code	Coverage Field	Statute	X-Ref	PI	ASC Pay Grp
C1012	PLATELET CONCENTRATE, LEUKOREDUCED, IRRADIATED, EACH UNIT	D	D	1833(T)	P9033	53	
C1013	PLATELET CONCENTRATE, LEUKOREDUCED, EACH UNIT	D	D	1833(T)	P9031	53	
C1014	PLATELET, LEUKOREDUCED, APHERESIS/PHERESIS, EACH UNIT	D	D	1833(T)	P9035	53	

As you can see by looking at the example, the code C1012 stands for a platelet concentrate. You will notice that the pricing index is 53 which means (according to the chart above), that the code would not be paid by Medicare. (You know this because 53 stands for statute and as was mentioned before, there are things that are either covered or non-covered by Medicare statute.) Additionally, in this case there is other information that supports the fact that C1012 is not covered. For example, when we look at both the Action Code field and the Coverage field you can see the notation D (under Action Code) which tells you that the code has been "Discontinued" and D under the Coverage field which stands for the fact that special coverage instructions apply, both meaning that the code would not have been covered by Medicare statute.

hint

Be sure to read all of the fields and see how they interplay with one another. The notations in all the fields are important to look at ***in unison.***

ASC Payment Group

If you are coding for an ASC (ambulatory surgery center), you will need this field as it will describe what payment group the code you have selected will fall into and, likewise, the amount of money that your facility will be reimbursed. The following is a list of the notations and the corresponding dollar amounts that you will see in the **2003 HCPCS National Coding Manual**. (This list was last updated in October, 2000.)

ACS Payment Group	
Group 1	$323
Group 2	$433
Group 3	$495
Group 4	$612
Group 5	$696
Group 6	$806*
Group 7	$966
Group 8	$949*

*$150 of the amount allowed in these two groups is for the intraocular lenses.

Below you will see an example in the Group 2 ASC Payment Group. This was the only ASC Payment Group code that we could find throughout the government's version of the **2003 HCPCS National Coding Manual**.

HCPC	Long Description	Action Code	Coverage Field	Statute	X-Ref	PI	ASC Pay Grp
G0105	COLORECTAL CANCER SCREENING; COLONOSCOPY ON INDIVIDUAL AT HIGH RISK	N	D			11	02

Why there are no others groups (besides the Group 2 notation) in the **HCPCS National Coding Manual** at this time is unknown to me. One would surmise that the other groups have not yet been assigned.

Summary

CHAPTER THREE

- ✓ There are many fields given for HCPCS National codes, eight of which are particularly important to the coder.
- ✓ The HCPCS field gives you the number of the actual code or modifier.
- ✓ The Coverage Field gives information on whether or not a code is covered.
- ✓ The Action Code field describes what has happened to the code (e.g., what Medicare has done to it as in adding, deleting or changing it).
- ✓ The Statute field which tells the coder if the code is not covered by Medicare statute.
- ✓ The ASC Payment Group field gives information on how much the supply, procedure or service is "worth". NOTE: Only the ASC Payment Group 2 is listed in the 2003 version of HCPCS National Codes.
- ✓ The X-Ref field tells you that another code has been substituted for the one you are using.

✓ The Price Indicator (PI) field tells you how Medicare arrives at the fee for the service, supply or procedure.

✓ The Processing Notes field explains additional information that the carriers take into account in processing a code. Processing Notes can be found at the nd of your **HCPCS National Coding Manual.**

CHAPTER FOUR

CPT: FORMAT OF THE BOOK

CPT is built on sets of numerical codes that identify procedures and services in six separate sections: Evaluation and Management, Anesthesia, Surgery, Radiology, Pathology and Laboratory, and Medicine. The formats of these sections are similar in that they all feature guidelines and other helpful hints that provide ground rules for using the chapters.

CPT is composed of a system of five-digit numeric codes. Following is an example of a **CPT** code:

99201 *Office or other outpatient visit for the evaluation and management of a new patient, which requires these three key components:*

- *a problem-focused history;*
- *a problem-focused exam; and*
- *straightforward medical decision-making.*

Counseling and/or coordination of care with other providers or agencies are provided consistent with the nature of the problem(s) and the patient's and/or family's needs.

Usually, the presenting problem(s) are self-limited or minor. Physicians typically spend 10 minutes face-to-face with the patient and/or family.

As you can see, this code has five digits:

Code:	**9**	**9**	**2**	**0**	**1**
Digits:	*1*	*2*	*3*	*4*	*5*

No two codes in **CPT** are alike; each means something different. That is, each code is used only once in the book to describe a specific procedure, service, or supply. A code may be deleted because (a) the procedure or service the code describes has been changed or is no longer being performed by physicians, or (b) the code describing the procedure has been replaced by another code. In either case, the number used for that code will not be reused if at all possible. This means that your office will not run the risk of getting paid for an obsolete procedure or service (which

No two codes are alike...

could be a problem if the practice is audited). You may have to pay back any money that the IRS feels you shouldn't have received. For this reason, you need to keep abreast of all changes made each year.

Because the codes and descriptors are updated, revised, or changed as needed, it is important that you change your own coding scheme each year. If your office uses a superbill or preprinted routing slip that lists your procedures, it is critical that you update this form each year.

A Look Through the Book

In the first few pages of **CPT** following the foreword, you will find a listing of the AMA CPT editorial panel. These are the people who implement suggestions and changes for the next year's volume of **CPT**. The editorial panel decides whether the additions and changes suggested by physicians and their staffs, insurance carriers, medical associations, or people like you would, in fact, make the next version of the **CPT** book better than the last.

The AMA CPT advisory committee is listed in the book following the editorial panel. Members of this committee are selected by their colleagues to represent each of their respective specialties.

The responsibilities of physicians on the AMA CPT advisory committee include answering questions directed to them from the AMA CPT editorial panel about a particular code, as well as assisting the editorial panel in determining the appropriateness of a particular revision or addition to **CPT**.

Although there will never be enough space to list all of the persons responsible for the success of **CPT**, without the help and support of people like you, the book would never be as complete as it is.

Following the advisory committee listing, you will find the AMA's Health Care Professionals advisory committee (HCPAC). This is a group pf people that, like the CPT advisory committee, have also been selected by the particular organizations that they represent (e.g., American Occupational Therapy Association, American Psychological Association). Note that this group of people represent health care fields (e.g., dieticians, nurses, social workers) who are not medical doctors (non-M.D.'s). The input of these groups is critical in the overall continued development of **CPT** in that the services they provide impact the overall health care of the patients they serve. Likewise, some of the procedures found in **CPT** represent services that these individuals (and individuals like them) perform.

It is easy to see that, excluding the introduction, Category III codes and the appendices, the **CPT** book is divided into six major sections:

1. Evaluation and Management
2. Anesthesia
3. Surgery
4. Radiology
5. Pathology and Laboratory
6. Medicine

These sections will be discussed in detail later. At this point, it is enough to know that each section has its own numbering system and that each (as implied by the names of the sections) has its own unique kinds of procedures and services.

Each Section Has A Numbering System

As we said earlier, the first digit in each **CPT** code begins with a number from 0 through 9.

Evaluation and Management heads up the main part of **CPT**. Codes in this section begin with the number 9 and describe the different histories, examinations, supervision of patients, and decisions physicians must make in evaluating and treating patients in a variety of settings (e.g., office/outpatient, hospital).

The types of procedures and services described in the Evaluation and Management Section are those that were found previously in the Medicine Section under "Levels of Service." Because of the government's Omnibus Budget Reconciliation Act (OBRA) of 1989 and its goal of achieving a balanced budget, HCFA, now called CMS, implemented the resource-based relative value study, conducted by researchers at Harvard University. This study suggested that it was impossible to arrive at the cost of individual physician procedures and services using the Levels of Service codes. It was discovered that physicians were not using these codes consistently and that a more accurate measure needed to be developed to describe more precisely the procedures and services that they were providing to their patients.

To solve this problem, the AMA — in conjunction with HCFA produced the Evaluation and Management Section. This section accounted for the type of history taken, the type of examination performed, and the level of decision-making required to diagnose and treat the patient.

Codes in the next section of **CPT**, Anesthesia, begin with the number 0. The Anesthesia Section is not always used by carriers since there is a conflict between the numbering system used here and the previous system chosen by the American Dental Association to code dental procedures and services. It is important that you contact your carrier beforehand to verify how you should be coding for anesthesia procedures. (For example, should you use Surgery codes with other notations known as "modifiers" to denote anesthesia procedures, or should you use the codes in the Anesthesia section?)

Modifiers for the Anesthesia Section can be found in a variety of places, depending on the carrier to which the claim is submitted. A great number of modifiers for Anesthesia are found at the beginning of the **National Coding Manual**.

As you learned in Chapter Two, except for Evaluation and Management, the first digits used for codes in the sections occur in the order in which the sections are presented. All codes in the Anesthesia Section (with the exception of some codes known as "Qualifying Circumstances for Anesthesia and others for sedation") begin with 0, in the Surgery Section with 1 through 6, in the Radiology Section with 7, in the Pathology and Laboratory Section with 8, and in the Medicine Section with 9. Each of these will be discussed in detail in the following chapters.

Although knowing which numbers are found in each section may sound elementary at first, remembering the arrangement is one of the most important things you can do to make coding easier. It is the first digit that will assist you in determining the correctness of a code.

hint

In short, the arrangement of the sections and the numbering system of each can be described in the following way:

SECTION	FIRST DIGIT
Evaluation and Management	*9*
Anesthesia	*0*
Surgery	*1 through 6*
Radiology	*7*
Pathology and Laboratory	*8*
Medicine	*9*

To illustrate this point, let's consider the following example. Suppose you were to review a claim filed by one of your co-workers. On the claim, your co-worker entered "88910 Telephone call."

By knowing that a telephone call is a noninvasive procedure and not a special pathology or lab test, you would know before even checking your **CPT** book that the code was incorrect, i.e., that the number 8 is found only in the Pathology and Laboratory Section and that the telephone call should have begun with the number 9.

Let's consider another example. Let's say you were a consultant reviewing the superbill of your client. On the form, you found a code listed that read "63020 Radiologic Exam, shoulder."

Instantly you would realize that the correct code begins with the number 7, because **all** Radiology codes begin with the number 7, and that use of this code for a shoulder x-ray is incorrect.

CPT Introduction: A Handy Reference Tool

Following the table of contents is the Introduction, one of the handiest reference tools the coder can use.

In the introduction you will find the insights and rules that were used in organizing **CPT**. Instructions for use of the book are given here, as well as the layout of procedures and codes. The introduction also includes an explanation of modifiers, a description of unlisted procedures and services, editorial notations, and information on CD-ROM and computer disks that are available to you. For more information on CD-ROM and diskettes call (800) 621-8335.

If you have not already read the introduction to the **CPT** book, it is important that you do so.

More Reference Tools in Each Section

Following the introduction are the six major sections of the book, each of which begins with its own guidelines.

The guidelines may contain several things: a definition of terms used in that section, an explanation of the notes that appear in and around different codes, a listing of the unlisted procedures found throughout that particular section, an explanation of how to file a special report, and a list of all modifiers appropriate for use in that particular section. You may also find definitions that will assist you with different words and phrases you will encounter throughout the section (e.g., new patient and established patient).

Following the guidelines is the body of the section. It is here that the actual codes and their descriptions can be found.

You will see that the code numbers in **CPT** are listed in numerical order. (The exception is the Evaluation and Management Section that heads up the book and whose codes begin with the number 9.) This is not significant from a payment standpoint. In other words, it is not correct to assume that just because the number is higher (in numeric sequence), the payment also will be higher (although reimbursement sometimes seems to work that way).

Category III Codes

The Category III codes were a new addition to the **CPT** book for 2002. These codes are alphanumeric (that is, they contain a letter of the alphabet and four other numbers) but are different from the HCPCS National Codes in that the alpha character (the letter) comes after the numbers instead of before. So far, the Category III codes range from

0001T through 00044T. The Category III codes are currently listed in numerical order as opposed to an order placed by a particular body part (e.g., musculoskeletal system) or kind of service (e.g., Evaluation and Management) The kinds of services listed in the Category III codes are mixed up. That is, you will not find a grouping of all codes that have to do with OB/GYN together. They may be interspersed throughout the total grouping of Category III codes.

Let's look at some examples of Category III codes:

0003T *Cervicography*

0005T *Transcatheter placement of extracranial cerebrovascular artery stent(s), percutaneous; initial vessel*

0009T *Endometrial cryoablation with ultrasonic guidance*

As you can see, the numbers begin with zero and the digits end with a "T." The "T" means the codes are temporary. That is, they have been placed in the **CPT** book for some period of time (an unspecified period of time) by the AMA. These codes are available for use by the physician or clinician in place of the unlisted procedure codes (those that almost always end in the number "99" (e.g., 68899) and are found at the end of each subsection in **CPT**). There may be instances in which you feel that the temporary code is the best choice for coding a procedure that you do. Remember that you can use these whenever they apply.

The temporary codes are available to measure emerging technology, find out if in fact physicians are using these procedures and whether or not an actual code assignment (and non-temporary code) needs to be added to either the **CPT** book or the **HCPCS National Coding Manual**. Because these codes are temporary, reflect emerging technology found in medicine and will be archived after five years if trends do not prove that physicians are in fact providing these services, the AMA has decided to make new Category III codes available (as they are released) through their internet-site via the AMA/**CPT** web site. The AMA will publish a complete list of the Category III codes every year with the release of the new **CPT** book.

APPENDICES: NOT A SECTION TO OVERLOOK!

Following the six sections and the Category III codes are the appendices.

Appendix A features a complete listing of modifiers found throughout the book, although modifiers that apply to each particular section are also found at the beginning of each section. You will also find HCPCS Level II modifiers in Appendix A as well as modifiers approved for ambulatory surgical centers and the anesthesia physical status modifiers. Each of these modifiers is used in a similar fashion to the way regular **CPT** modifiers are used. For a more comprehensive discussion on modifiers found in this appendix of

CPT, please refer to the chapter on Modifiers. The HCPCS Level II modifiers are self-explanatory.

Appendix B is a summary of the additions, deletions, and revisions that have been made to the book during the year. By using this appendix, you will find it easy to update your superbill, encounter form, or master coding sheet without having to look through the entire book, as long as you do so on an annual basis.

Revisions of the **CPT** book can be purchased from the AMA in both diskette (long version with the complete code and description and short version with the procedure outlined in 28 or fewer characters) and CD-ROMs.

For the vast majority of coders, the use of Appendix B, together with use of the body of the book for reference purposes, is adequate for updating codes.

Appendix C was formerly a summary of additions deletions and revisions just like Appendix B. This was because the AMA used to have to distinguish between changes that happened on their "short description tape" and changes on their "long or full description tape". (Most of this was necessary for the big main-frame computers that had to have "tapes". Nowadays with the use of personal computers and others that require different types of input (e.g., diskettes or CD Roms') the use of the "tapes" is virtually obsolete. Because of this, the Appendix C for revisions, deletions and additions of tapes is now an appendix which contains examples of many of the levels of service found in the Evaluation and Management Section (the codes that begin with 9). It is here that you can verify whether or not you are coding the evaluation and management services correctly. It is important to remember, however, that just because an example may seem the same as the case of a patient you are seeing, it does *not* necessarily mean that you must code your patient's claim in that way. This will be discussed further in the chapter on Evaluation and Management.

Appendix D is a list of the add-on codes found in **CPT**. Add-on codes are those that should be listed (if appropriate) in addition to the code for the main service.

An example would be the following:

*11200** *Removal of skin tags, multiple fibrocutaneous tags, any area; up to and including 15 lesions*

✚ *11201* *each additional ten lesions (list separately in addition to code for primary procedure).*

Note that the 11201 is an "add-on" code to be used "in addition" to the code 11200 (the first 15 lesions), when a patient has 20 lesions for example.

Appendix E lists a summary of the **CPT** codes that do not require the use of the modifier -51 (Multiple Procedures). Multiple procedures will be discussed further in "Chapter Eleven: Modifiers."

THE INDEX

As the name **CPT (Current Procedural Terminology)** implies, the first thing you should do when trying to locate a code is look in the index for the "procedure" or "service" performed. For example, let's suppose your physician performed a surgical arthroscopy on a patient's elbow. The procedure in this case is arthroscopy. Looking up the code in the index for arthroscopy, you would see the following:

Arthroscopy
Diagnostic
Elbow 29830
Hip 29860
Knee 29870
Metacarpophalangeal joint 29900
Shoulder 29805
Surgical
Ankle .... 29891 - 29899
Elbow .... 29834 - 29838

Because you are looking for surgical arthroscopy on the elbow, you would select the entry that says "Surgical, Elbow, 29834-29838." You will note that a range of codes is given. That is, the book tells you to look for any code within a set of numbers (e.g., 29834-29838, Surgical, Elbow). It would be important, at this point, to look up the range of codes in the text and select the code which most closely describes the procedure you have just performed.

The "range" concept is different from what you will find in most books where the index cites a page number or numbers on which a particular item can be found. In **CPT,** the page number is not cited. Rather, the range of codes that includes the procedure or service is given. Knowing that the book is arranged in numeric order, beginning with 9 for Evaluation and Management and followed by everything else from 0 through 9, it is easy to locate the page(s) where the code will be found.

Let's take another example. Let's say you were looking for an arthroscopy performed on the elbow for *diagnostic* purposes. In this case, you would see that the book only lists one code for you to look at—that being 29830.

Sometimes a procedure, service, or supply is not listed in the index and must be found by a different means. Another way is to look it up by the body organ or anatomic site involved. Let's say, for example, the procedure provided to the patient was the repair of a femur fracture.

The list in the index under "femur" (the anatomic site in this case), includes the following:

Femur

...

...

...

Repair 27470-27472

Epiphysis 27181, 27475, 27742

Another way to find a code is to look under the condition for which the patient is being treated. For example, does the patient have tumors or adhesions? By looking up the suggested code ranges, you would be able to locate the appropriate repair code.

Let's suppose the patient has eye adhesions. Looking up "Adhesions" in the index, you would find the following:

Adhesions
Eye...
Corneovitreal...*65880*
Incision
Anterior Segment .... *65860 - 65870*
Posterior Segment *65875*

From the list, you would be able to find the adhesion for which you were trying to bill, as well as the range of codes in which the procedure was located.

Another example:

Suppose the patient had an abscess of the abdomen. If you were to look up this condition (abscess), you would find the following:

Abscess
Abdomen. .... *49040 - 49041*
Incision & Drainage
Open.. *49040*
Percutaneous *49021*

If you have been unsuccessful in locating a procedure or code in one of the ways mentioned above, try looking up the procedure, organ, or condition in your dictionary to find a synonym for it. For example, if you need a code for something having to do with cancer, you might look up the procedure or code under "carcinoma." Or, if you need a code for something concerning the heart, you might also check under "cardiac."

It is also important to check under eponyms. An eponym in **CPT** is the use of a person's name to describe a condition, procedure, or service. Examples are the Colles Fracture or Marshall-Marchetti-Krantz Procedure. Both of these can be found under the proper names of their inventors.

The last way to find a procedure is by looking up its abbreviation. Code ranges for most procedures that are commonly abbreviated can be found in this manner. For example, you may need to find a code for the creatine phosphokinase test. By checking under "CPK" in the index, you would find the appropriate range of codes (82550-82552). In cases to which this does not apply, you may have to find out what an abbreviation stands for and look up the entire word. The use of a good abbreviation dictionary can greatly assist you with this task.

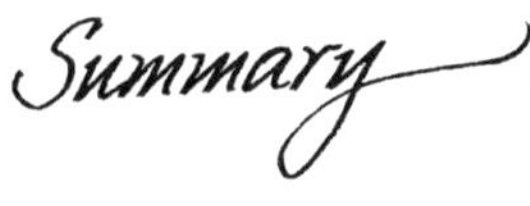

CHAPTER FOUR

- ✓ **CPT** is composed of a system of five-digit numeric codes.
- ✓ **CPT** is updated annually.
- ✓ The coder needs to keep abreast of changes made each year to **CPT**.
- ✓ The seven major sections of **CPT** and their numeric headers:

Section	**First Digit**
Evaluation and Management	9
Anesthesia	0
Surgery	1 through 6
Radiology	7
Pathology and Laboratory	8
Medicine	9
Category III	0

- ✓ Knowing the numeric headers can help you find a mistake on your claim form, master sheet, or superbill.
- ✓ Incorrect codes = incorrect information.
- ✓ The introduction of **CPT** is important.
- ✓ Guidelines preceding a section give the ground rules for that section.
- ✓ Category III codes are temporary codes that help measure and identify emerging services.
- ✓ Category III codes are found before the appendices toward the back of the **CPT** book.
- ✓ Category III codes (if available) should be used in place of unlisted procedures.
- ✓ Appendix A is a complete list of all available modifiers.
- ✓ Appendix B is a summary of the additions, deletions, and revisions that have been made to the book for that year.

- ✓ Appendix C gives examples of the different kinds of Evaluation and Management codes.

- ✓ Appendix D lists the add-on codes that should be used in addition to the codes for the primary procedures when appropriate.

- ✓ Appendix E lists the codes that when used in conjunction with other codes do ***not*** require the addition of the modifier -51 (Multiple Procedures).

- ✓ The coder needs to be as resourceful as possible in looking up a code in the index.

CHAPTER FIVE

CPT: EDITORIAL NOTATIONS

In order to understand **CPT**, you must know how and why the book denotes or marks certain procedures.

hint

If you are coding for a hospital outpatient setting, be sure to get the appropriate ***CPT*** *book for hospital outpatient coding. Additional editorial notations are listed in that book that are not found in the regular version of* ***CPT*** *but are important to you from a coding and billing standpoint. You can find the* ***CPT 2003: Hospital Outpatient Services: A Specially Annotated Version for Use in Hospital Outpatient Settings*** *by logging onto several websites (e.g., MedBooks.com or 800 443-7397) or by calling the AMA directly at 800-621-8335.*

Six notations used in **CPT** for physician coding are important to understand. These are called editorial notations.

An editorial notation is a sign to the coder that something about a particular code is different from other codes in the book. When you see an editorial notation, you need to take care in using that code number.

Before going into detail on the six editorial notations, let's look at each of them:

●	the bullet
▲	the triangle
✱	the star (asterisk)
▸ ◂	double inverted triangles
✚	the plus sign
⊘	the exempt symbol

Now we will discuss each notation in detail, so you may understand why each is so important from a biller's perspective.

THE BULLET (●)

The bullet precedes the code and means that the code and its description are new to the book for that year.

Here is an example of the bullet in the 2003 **CPT** book:

● *99293 Initial pediatric critical care, 31 days up through 24 months of age, per day, for the evaluation and management of a critically ill infant or young child.*

An example of the bullet in the 2002 **CPT** book was:

● *33980 Removal of ventricular assist device, implantable intracorporeal, single ventricle*

Look in your current version of **CPT** for examples of bullets. Bullets appear for only one year and may be found in any section. They denote that the procedure before which they appear is a new procedure for that year.

hint

Bullet (●) = new code.

The bullet is important because it signals to the biller that the code was not found in the book the previous year. You should take special note because this code might be one you may have needed in the past.

THE TRIANGLE (▲)

The triangle precedes the code and means that the description of the code has changed since last year.

Here is an example of a ▲ from the 2003 **CPT** book:

▲ *11600 Excision, malignant lesion including margins, trunk, arms, or legs, excised diameter 0.5 cm or less*

The following is an example of a triangle from the 2002 **CPT** book:

▲ *33975 Insertion of ventricular assist device; extracorporeal, single ventricle*

Check in your version of **CPT** for examples of triangles. Like bullets, triangles appear for only one year and can be found in any section. They denote that the procedure before which they appear has been revised or changed in some way for the new volume of **CPT**.

hint

Triangle (▲) = revised code.

The triangle is important because it signals the biller that something has been revised or deleted from the description of the procedure and that the code description this year differs from last year's code description.

Although the difference may not appear great at first, the impact on reimbursement could be significant. You should compare the codes that have changed in the current version of **CPT** to those listed the previous year. Many times, when the description of the code has changed, the reimbursement has also been affected.

By not paying attention to the bullet and the triangle, you stand to lose money on reimbursement. Codes that have been deleted or revised, codes that no longer mean exactly what they meant last year, and codes that denote new procedures all have some bearing on how the procedure should be billed.

THE STAR (ASTERISK) (✱)

The star, or asterisk, is probably the notation that has the most immediate impact to the coder. Unlike the bullet or the triangle, the star follows a code. That is, it comes after the code in the right margin.

An example of the star is:

36415   Collection of venous blood by venipuncture*

hint

Star (✱) = Surgical Package concept does not apply.
The "a la carte" concept does apply.

The star means that the Surgical Package concept (see below) does not apply, and that you need to bill separately for the different components of the Surgical Package, if appropriate, in addition to billing for the starred procedure.

Stars can be found only in the Surgery Section of **CPT** (on codes beginning with the numbers 1, 2, 3, 4, 5, and 6). They will never be found in any other section. Because the star means that the surgical package concept does not apply (e.g., that the pre-op and post op services are NOT included with the procedure as listed) it stands to reason that you will only see stars on codes in the Surgery Section. In other words, you would not see a star on a service or procedure in any other section in **CPT** because none of the other sections have variable pre and post-operative services to begin with.

To explain this further, we need to understand the Surgical Package. If you've ever had lunch at a "50's diner" (or dinner, if you were ***really*** lucky), you may remember the "blue plate special." If you haven't been fortunate enough to dine there, perhaps you've eaten at another place that serves these specials. You will recall that "blue plate specials" include everything = the roast beef, baked potato, string beans, drink, etc. - for one low price. In other words, you get a "package deal."

For those of you who have taken a slightly fancier approach to dining, you may have had the pleasure of eating at a fine French restaurant where your menu was priced by the individual items you chose. For example, the appetizer was priced separately from the entree, the dessert, and so on. In other words, your menu was a la carte: you paid for each item separately. You probably paid more, too, but at least you had the flexibility of choosing a variety of items from the menu.

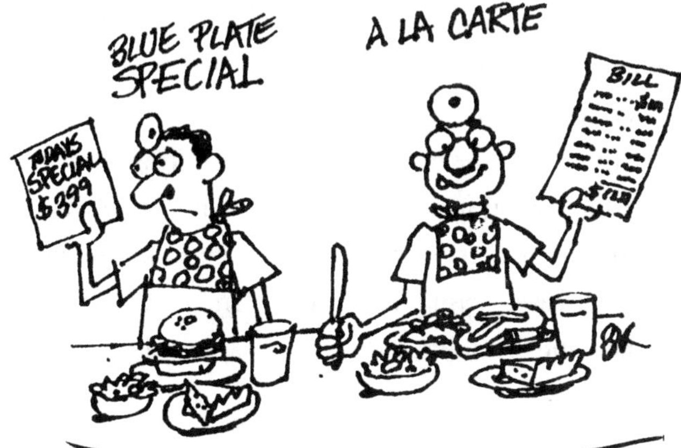

The surgical package resembles a "blue plate special" where everything is included in one price. Starred procedures are similar to an "a la carte" menu: everything is priced separately.

The concept of billing and coding for a starred procedure and its component parts is similar to the concept of ordering and paying for items from an a la carte menu. The price per item stays the same, but the overall grand total may differ, depending on what was requested.

The Surgical Package concept in **CPT** is similar to the "blue plate special" in the way it is coded and billed. Likewise, starred surgical procedures are similar to the a la carte menu. According to both the AMA and the CMS (Center for Medicare and Medicaid Services, who administers the Medicare program), the Surgical Package includes pre-op, surgery and post-op, whereas starred surgical services (a la carte) do not include all of the above. Instead, the procedures and services are priced separately.

The **CPT** manual defines the surgical package to include local infiltration, metacarpal digital block, or topical anesthesia, when used, the E/M service (directly related to the surgery) on the day of or the day before the surgery (it does not include the visit during which you decided to operate), the operation per se, and normal, uncomplicated follow-up care including the discussion with the family, checking the patient in post-anesthesia recovery, writing note and orders, and discussion with the family. Schematically, this **CPT** Surgical Package looks like the following:

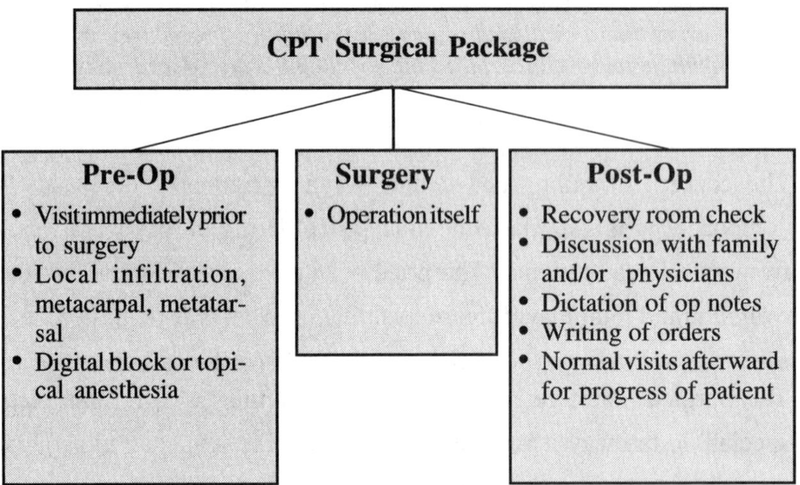

In 1992, the definition of the Surgical Package for Medicare changed to include any related services including the history exam and medical decision-making (pre-op) performed no more than one day prior to surgery, the operation per se, and normal, uncomplicated follow-up care (from 0 to 90 days). The initial evaluation or consultation by the surgeon in which the decision to operate is made is not included in the Surgical

Package and will be paid separately. You may be required by your carrier to use the modifier -57 on the end of this initial evaluation to indicate that it was not part of the global-fee period (e.g., that this was the visit during which you decided to operate). For more information on modifiers, read Chapter Eleven.

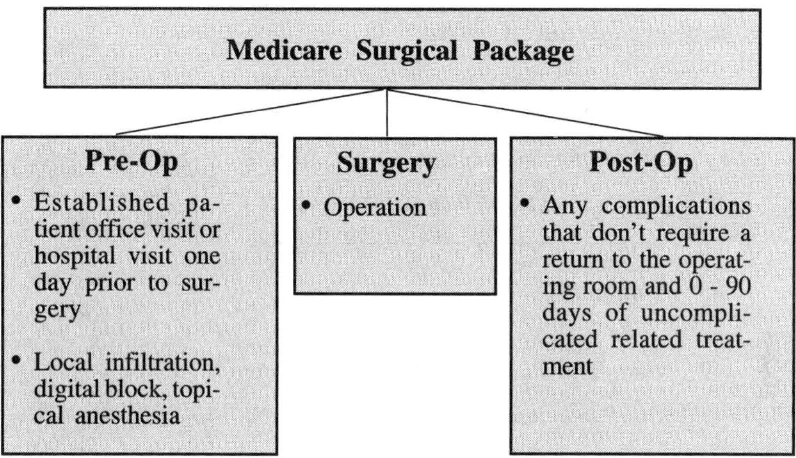

As you view the diagrams, the two Surgical Packages (AMA's and Medicare's) look pretty much the same. The difference between the two Surgical Packages can be confusing to the coder but lies mainly in the nuances surrounding the post-op care (i.e., Medicare says post-op ranges from zero through ninety days and the AMA does not define post-op in that way. This nuance will be discussed in greater detail in the chapter on Surgery).

When you see a procedure followed by the star (✱), you should note that the Surgical Package concept (everything included in one price) does **not** apply. Because the Surgical Package concept does not hold true for starred procedures, you must complete it by adding (coding) the pre-op and post-op services provided.

Certain rules for starred procedures are listed in the guidelines of the Surgery Section of your **CPT** book. It is important that we review these and, that you as a coder, have a complete understanding of them. For the time being, note the following:

1. Starred procedures will be found only in the section on Surgery. This makes sense, as stars are found on procedures that need to have a Surgical Package completed.

2. Usually, smaller surgical procedures that have indefinite pre-ops and post-ops are those that are starred.

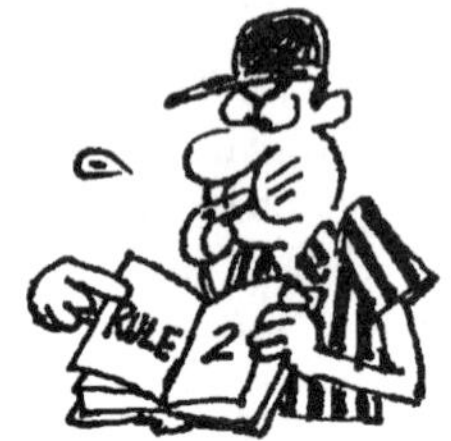

What do we mean by "indefinite pre-ops and post-ops" in rule 2? To illustrate an indefinite pre-op or post-op for a small surgical procedure, let's consider the following example.

Suppose you work for a dermatologist. A patient comes into your office with an abscess the size of a nickel. Before aspirating the abscess, the dermatologist completes an exam obtaining such information as the patient's complaint. The exam also includes a complete study of the integumentary (skin) system as it applies to this abscess, during which the doctor asks the patient some questions about the origin of the lesion. She then cleanses the wound and aspirates the lesion. The dermatologist places a bandage on the lesion to keep it from becoming infected and prescribes an antibiotic.

Your insurance person places the following information on the claim form:

> *10160** *Puncture aspiration of abscess, hematoma, bulla or cyst*
>
>

As you can see, the code adequately describes the puncture aspiration of the abscess, even though it does not describe its extent (benign). It also does not describe the history, exam, or decision toward treatment that occurred before the actual aspiration.

A week or so later, this same patient calls your office to say that the site of the lesion looks very red and is tender to the touch. When questioned, the patient admits that he has not taken any antibiotics nor has he kept the lesion very clean. You ask the patient to return for a follow-up visit.

The next day, another patient comes into your office complaining of an abscess. This time, the abscess is approximately the size of a "clicker," or the end of a ballpoint pen.

Your doctor examines the abscess and decides to aspirate. She cleanses the lesion with alcohol, aspirates it, places the patient on antibiotics and advises him to contact her if he has any further problems.

Your biller places the following on the claim form:

10160 Puncture aspiration of abscess, hematoma, bulla or cyst*

Think about the two scenarios presented above. What's different about them? Did you notice that the pre-op (that which happened before the surgery) in the first case was much more involved than the history and physical that occurred in the second case? Did you notice that the post-op (that which happened after the surgery) in the first case was also much more involved than in the second case? The patient in the second case does not necessarily need to return for a follow-up visit. In the first case, the patient needs to return for review of the lesion because it appears to be infected.

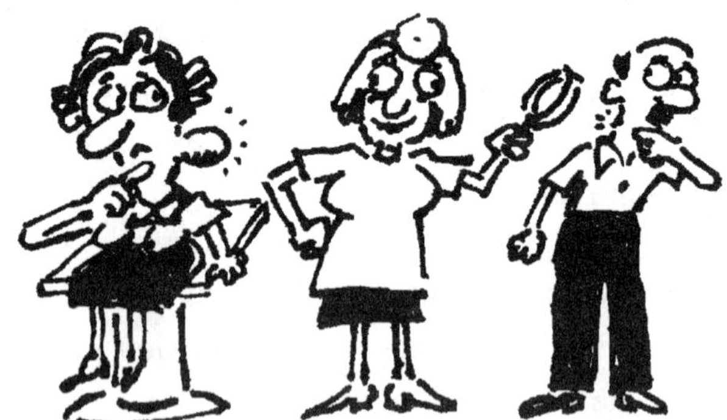

A visual comparison of the Surgical Package. The case on the left is much more involved because of the nature of the wound.

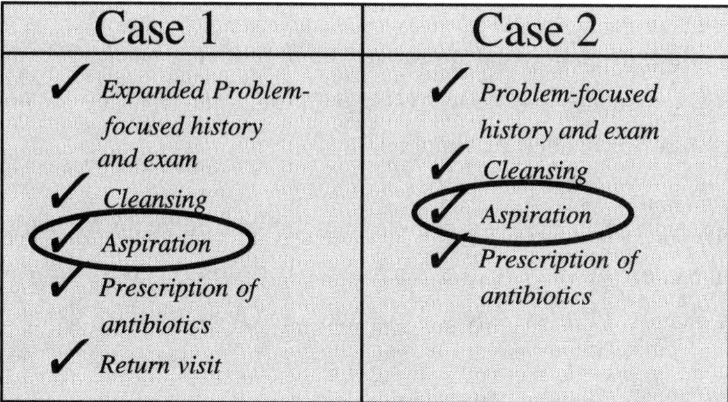

Upon examination, it is easy to see that the main part of the procedure listed above remained constant while everything that happened before and after the surgery was variable.

Because the extent of pre-op and post-op care cannot be predicted in real life, the **CPT** editorial panel and the **CPT** advisory committee decided to denote procedures such as these with a star. The star calls the coder's attention to the fact that the Surgical Package is incomplete and gives the coder the flexibility of adding the appropriate pre-op and post-op services provided.

CPT lists four basic rules for the coding of starred procedures. We will examine each of these rules in detail in the Surgery Section under Starred (✱) Procedures or Items.

For the time being, let's just say that when you see a starred procedure, you need to think about completing the Surgical Package by adding appropriate codes (if indicated) to the claim form.

THE INVERTED TRIANGLES (▸ ◂)

This editorial notation first appeared in **CPT** 1998. The inverted triangles show the reader that some text other than the actual descriptions of the codes has been added or changed.

An example of the inverted triangles can be found under the Musculoskeletal System in Surgery, (see Endoscopy/Arthroscopy page 100, 2003 **CPT** Standard Edition, second Column), and read as follows:

- ▸ *(For open or mini-open rotator cuff repair, use 23412)* ◂
- ▸ *(When arthroscopic subacromial decompression is performed at the same setting, use 29826 and append modifier –51)* ◂

Note that one inverted triangle comes before the phrase and the other comes at the end of the phrase.

The inverted triangles will only appear before and after the verbiage for one year and can be found anywhere in the **CPT** book.

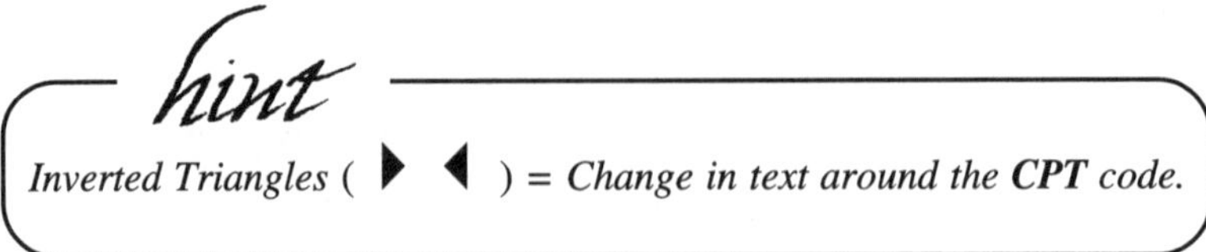

hint
Inverted Triangles (▸ ◂) = Change in text around the ***CPT*** *code.*

THE PLUS SIGN (✚)

Codes that have the plus sign are known as "add-on codes." You will find some services in **CPT** that take into account "more parts" of another service. Consider the following example:

*11200** *Removal of skin tags, multiple fibrocutaneous tags, any area; up to and including 15 lesions.*

✚ *11201* *each additional ten lesions (List separately in addition to code for primary procedure)*

As you can see, the 11201 describes each additional ten lesions and this code needs to be listed *in addition to* the code for the 11200. Add-on codes let the coder know that if you are trying to describe the greater extent of the service (e.g., that there were more parts that you did than described in the original service) you will need both codes (maybe even more than that depending on the service) to describe the entire procedure.

hint

The Plus Sign (✚) = Additional work associated with the main service.

Add-on codes are additional or supplemental procedures that are "added onto" the original service if additional services are performed at the same time as the initial service. These can be readily identified in the description of the code because the description uses words like "each additional" or "list separately in addition to the primary procedure."

The add-on code concept applies only to procedures performed by the same physician. For example, if one doctor performed the removal of skin tags above (11200*) and removed fifteen lesions and another doctor removed an additional ten, each doctor would use the code 11200 to account for the services. Note that even though a total 25 lesions were removed from the patient, the second ten lesions were removed by a different doctor and, therefore, were not subject to the add-on concept.

A summary of all add-on codes can be found in Appendix D of the **CPT** book.

Add-on codes do not require the use of the Multiple Procedures modifier -51, which will be discussed in greater detail in Chapter Eleven.

hint

Because of the nature of what "add-on" codes mean (e.g., that they are extensions of the main service) they do not require the use of the modifier –51.

THE EXEMPT SYMBOL (⦸)

The exempt symbol in **CPT** specifically relates the fact that codes found with this notation do not require the use of the Multiple Procedure modifier -51.

An example of the exempt symbol on a **CPT** code is the following.

⦸ *22841 Internal spinal fixation by wiring of spinous process*

As of the writing of this book, **CPT** has given no explanation for why you would not need a modifier -51 on Multiple Procedures performed during the same session.

Summary

CHAPTER FIVE

- ✓ Six editorial notations in **CPT** for physician billing are the bullet, the triangle, the star, the inverted triangles, the plus sign and the exempt symbol.
- ✓ The bullet precedes (comes before) a code and means that the code and its associated description are new to the book for that year.
- ✓ Bullets can be found in any section of **CPT**.
- ✓ The triangle precedes a code and means that the description of the code has changed since last year.
- ✓ Triangles can be found in any section of **CPT**.
- ✓ Both bullets and triangles are found before a given code for only one year.

- ✓ The star follows a procedure code and means that the procedure for which you are billing does not include the pre-op and post-op services.

- ✓ Stars are found only after procedure codes in the Surgery Section—that is, codes beginning with the numbers 1, 2, 3, 4, 5, and 6.

- ✓ A star remains on a procedure code as long as the AMA **CPT** Editorial Panel feels that the procedure is a minor surgical procedure with an indefinite pre-op and post-op.

- ✓ In coding a starred procedure, the coder should make an additional effort to complete the Surgical Package by adding appropriate codes necessary to describe pre-op and post-op services.

- ✓ The inverted triangles (43) found before and after "phrases" (not **CPT** code descriptions) in the **CPT** book indicate new or revised text.

- ✓ Inverted triangles only appear for one year.

- ✓ Inverted triangles can be found in any section of **CPT**.

✓ The plus sign (✚) can be found year after year and may be located in any section of **CPT**.

✓ The plus sign (✚) indicates that additional work is associated with the main service (e.g., additional digit(s), lesion(s), etc.)

✓ Add-on codes are always performed in addition to the primary procedure and must never be reported as stand-alone services.

✓ You would not use the multiple procedures modifier -51 on an add-on code because it is already understood that these "add-on" services go in addition to the main service performed.

✓ The exempt symbol (⃠) means that you are not supposed to use the multiple procedures modifier -51 on the code preceded with this symbol.

CHAPTER SIX

EVALUATION AND MANAGEMENT

Now that we have completed a general study of the **CPT** book, it's time to review the manual section by section. As pointed out previously, **CPT** lists the Evaluation and Management Section first. The reason for this is that most coders use this section more than any other.

All codes in the Evaluation and Management Section begin with the number 9.

Four editorial notations will be found in the Evaluation and Management Section: the bullet (●) for new codes, the triangle (▲) for revised descriptors, the inverted triangles (►◄) which indicate new or revised text, and the plus sign (✚) which indicates that there may be additional parts that can be added onto the primary service. Starred (✱)

procedures and the exempt symbol (⊘) will never be found in Evaluation and Management; Stars are only found in the Surgery Section (codes beginning with the numbers 1, 2, 3, 4, 5, and 6) because they indicate that the Surgical Package concept does not apply.

Before exploring the nuances of each subsection, let's examine some of the terms you will see in Evaluation and Management.

NEW VERSUS ESTABLISHED PATIENTS

According to **CPT**, a new patient is one who has not received any professional services within the past three years from a given physician or another physician of the same specialty who belongs to the same group practice. An established patient is one who **has** received *professional services* within the past three years from that physician or another one of the same specialty who belongs to the same group.

In the 2001 **CPT** book, the AMA defined "professional services" (referring to new and established patients) as those services that occur face-to-face, are rendered by a physician, and reported by a **CPT** code.

We are all well aware that "professional services" in other sections of **CPT** can be things like x-rays, pathology services, electrocardiograms, etc. – some of which may or may not be face to face. The definition of professional services in this Evaluation and Management chapter is trying to say that in order to qualify for a particular "level" of Evaluation and Management service, the patient and physician or other health care professional must be face-to-face with the patient.

As you already know, there is part of the new patient definition that requires that a patient is only new to a physician if he or she has not seen the physician or another physician of the same specialty and of the same group practice within the last three years. In some instances though, carriers will allow you to code for a new patient visit if the patient is new to the physician of the same group practice if the physician is of a different *subspecialty.* For example, both physicians may be ophthalmologists, but one may have a *sub*specialty of pediatric ophthalmology and the other may be a retinal specialist. Find out if the patient would be considered "new" on their first visit to the 2nd physician of the group because of the three-year time frame, or if, because they were seeing someone of the same specialty (even though the sub-specialties were different), they would be considered an "established patient."

In most instances, a case can be made that a patient to these two sub-specialists would be new to each physician because of the differences in the kinds of services, examinations, etc. that they would provide to the patient. It is, however, always better to be safe (by checking) than sorry.

VISIT CODES

Once you determine whether the patient is new or established, you must decide which Evaluation and Management code to use for the visit. In prior versions of **CPT** (1991 and before), visit codes described differing "levels of service" that could be used to report the kinds of encounters physicians had with their patients. The coder saw terms such as

“Minimal,” “Brief,” “Limited,” “Intermediate,” “Extended,” and “Comprehensive” and had to choose the term that most accurately depicted a particular patient/physician encounter.

After this terminology had been used for quite some time, studies were conducted on the use of the codes. For example, the studies asked which codes physicians used the most and whether all levels of service were coded equally. When the usage of the levels of service was plotted on a graph the results showed the higher-levels-of-service codes were chosen more often. (See the following graph.) Results of these studies showed the use of the levels-of-service terms to be so variable that improper and, in many cases, inequitable payments were being made to physicians.

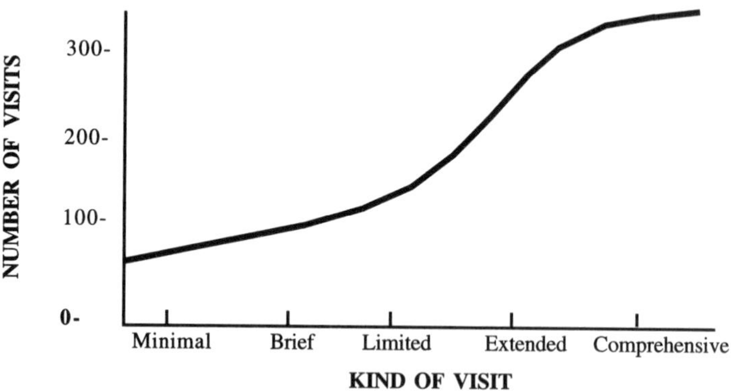

Largely due to the Omnibus Budget Reconciliation Act (OBRA) by which equitable payment and uniformity of payment among carriers across the nation were established by law, these codes and terms were changed.

The change helped establish factors and mathematical equations that could be used to determine how much a service was worth.

The final result was the Evaluation and Management codes. These codes, which replaced the old "level of service" codes, are very specific about what is or is not included in a particular visit. The following is an example of an Evaluation and Management code:

> *99201* *Office or other outpatient visit for the evaluation and management of a new patient, which requires these three key components:*
>
> - *a problem-focused history;*
> - *a problem-focused examination; and*
> - *straightforward medical decision-making.*
>
> *Counseling and/or coordination of care with other providers or agencies are provided consistent with the nature of the problem(s) and the patient's and/or family's needs.*
>
> *Usually, the presenting problem(s) are self-limited or minor. Physicians typically spend 10 minutes face-to-face with the patient and/or family.*

One of the best things you can do for your office is to keep in mind that Evaluation and Management ("E/M") codes deal with **what your physician does** during time spent with the patient rather than merely with the amount of time spent. By not paying attention to what is (or is not) included in each visit code, a biller can cost his or her physician a considerable amount of both time and money. Now more than ever before, it is critical for the physician to become involved in the decision as to which "E/M" code should be used for a specific patient/physician encounter. Without such input from the physician, it is impossible for any coder to accurately code these visits.

The entire Evaluation and Management Section is closely monitored by insurance carriers, but special emphasis has been placed on the following subsections:

- Office/Outpatient Services
- Hospital Inpatient Services
- Consultations (of all sorts)
- Emergency Department Services

As you examine the Evaluation and Management Section, you will see that many of the services described have something in common (e.g., they mention some sort of history, exam, and medical decision making). These are called "key components". To code levels of service accurately, you must be sure that two or three, depending on the category of the service, "key components" are present. Let's explain this in a little more detail.

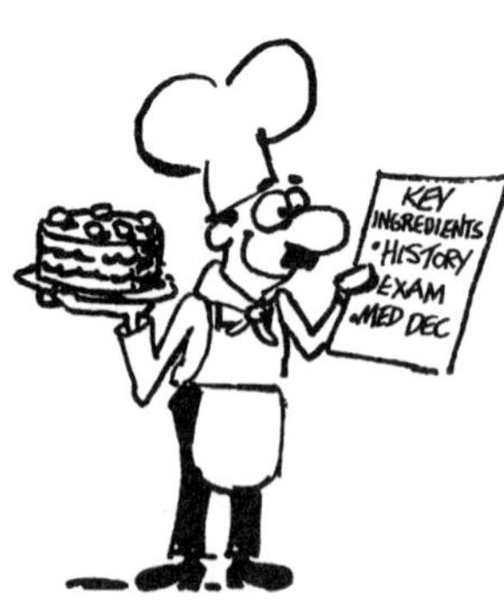

A "key component" is to a visit what an "important ingredient" is to a recipe.

A "key component" is to a visit what an "important or necessary ingredient" is to a recipe. For example, without the cheese, it isn't cheesecake. Likewise, without the "key components," it is not a visit.

Most Evaluation and Management codes contain the following general components (ingredients):

- history
- examination
- medical decision-making
- counseling
- coordination of care
- nature of presenting problem(s)
- time

However, not all of these are considered **key** components for the visit, just as vanilla extract, milk, and sour cream are not considered **key** ingredients for a cheesecake (at least not by me).

Key components for Evaluation and Management codes listed in **CPT** are the following:

- History (cheese)
- Examination (graham cracker crust)
- Medical decision-making (eggs)

When you take a look at the Evaluation and Management code on the preceding page (see 99201 for example), you can see the key ingredients that we are talking about. That is, you can see that the description of the code lists a kind of history, a kind of exam and a kind of medical decision making. Without these components, the service would not be considered an Evaluation and Management code.

Obviously, these key components vary from one service to another, and that's our next topic of discussion. Each key component will be explored individually.

When you refer back to this same code, 99201, on the preceding page of **CP"Teach"** you will see that some of the "terms" describing the different key components (e.g., problem-focused, expanded problem-focused) are used for both the history and examination. Don't be concerned about this, since the idea behind the terms is the same. What differs is the *action* that is taking place: whether the physician is taking a history or performing an examination.

A lot of people have great difficulty deciding which Evaluation and Management code to pick for the service they provide. It is easy to be intimidated by all of this material unless you realize that by slowly reading this book, we will walk you through the different kinds of Evaluation and Management services and by the time we are finished with this discussion and by the time we have given you the tools you need to be able to make the decision as to which level would be the appropriate choice, you will be close to being an expert. So take this discussion a page at a time and make sure that you understand each concept before proceeding to the next.

Remember: we will be putting all of these ideas together with the use of a special form (the DOC Form) which will help you consolidate your thoughts and the different components into a code selection that will appropriately describe the kind of Evaluation and Management service you provided to your patient. For right now, let's discuss each kind of history and exam.

Histories

As we said before, many of the Evaluation and Management services include main ingredients. These are the history(ies), theexam(s), and the medical decision making processes (e.g. what are we going to do to get this patient better). Each of these key ingredients will be discussed in detail.

Four kinds of histories are described in **CPT**:

- Problem-Focused History
- Expanded Problem-Focused History
- Detailed History
- Comprehensive History

If you have been coding for quite some time (1991 and before), you may think that the terms "detailed" and "comprehensive" sound familiar, and they should! Their definitions, however, are not the same for the new visit codes as they were for the "levels of service" codes used in previous versions of the book.

To increase your understanding of these terms, let's explore each of them separately.

Problem-Focused History

A problem-focused history is one in which the physician:

1. Obtains the chief complaint ("Why are you here today?");

   and

2. Takes a brief history of the present illness or problem.

The AMA's **CPT** book describes a chief complaint in the following way:

Chief Complaint: *"a concise statement describing the symptom, problem, con dition, diagnosis or other factor that is the reason for the encounter, usually stated in the patient's words."*

In summary then, a chief complaint is the reason the patient has come in — "Mrs. Jones, why are you here today?"

Obviously there will be times when the reason for the visit is more extensive than another. For example, the visit for someone who comes into your office following a car accident will be different from the visit for someone who needs an evaluation of itching.

It is not necessarily the chief complaint itself which will determine the kind of visit that follows. For example, someone may come into your office complaining of pain when he writes, and your history and exam may reveal a very serious problem (e.g., thoracic outlet syndrome). Notice that the chief complaint (minor arm pain) seems small in comparison to what the actual diagnosis turned out to be (thoracic outlet syndrome).

A problem-focused history is the kind your physician would take from a patient who comes in with a rash that looks like poison ivy. This kind of history might be taken if an out-of-town patient needs a prescription refilled. The physician focuses on the problem at hand. That is, he or she is not necessarily concerned with the fact that the patient may have (in addition to the rash) a broken leg or diabetes.

Questions your physician may ask as part of a problem-focused history include, but are not limited to, the following:

- What is the problem?
- How long have you had this problem?
- Are you taking any medications?
- Are you allergic to anything as far as you know?

Problem-focused histories are the simplest form of histories that can be taken.

Expanded Problem-Focused History

An expanded problem-focused history goes a little further than the problem-focused one. As its name implies, this type of history is expanded or enlarged so that the physician obtains more information than he did in the problem-focused history. In an expanded problem-focused history, the physician:

1. Obtains the chief complaint (like he did in the problem-focused history);
2. Takes a brief history of the present illness or problem; and
3. Conducts a problem-pertinent “system” review.

Let’s describe what a problem-pertinent system review is and how this makes an expanded problem-focused history different from a problem-focused history.

“Systems” that may receive the problem-pertinent system review include:

a. Eyes
b. Ears, nose, mouth and throat (ENT)
c. Cardiovascular
d. Respiratory
e. Gastrointestinal
f. Genitourinary
g. Musculoskeletal
h. Skin and/or breast (integumentary)
i. Neurologic
j. Psychiatric
k. Hematologic/Lymphatic/Immunologic/Allergic
l. Endocrine
m. Constitutional symptoms (fever, weight loss, etc.)

Your physician would take this kind of history from a male patient who comes in with severe cystic acne (e.g., skin or integumentary system) because the acne affects the integumentary system and may impact more than one body part (e.g., it is "expanded" to include head, neck and shoulders), or from a female child with a sore throat and headache (ENT and possible neurologic systems), which obviously affect more than one body part but are still relatively simple to diagnose and treat.

Questions your physician may ask as part of an expanded problem-focused history include, but are not limited to, the following:

- What is the problem?
- How long have you had this problem?
- Are you taking any medications?
- Are you allergic to anything as far as you know?
- Do you know what may be contributing to your problem?
- Are you experiencing this problem anywhere else?

Detailed History

In a detailed history, the physician does the following:

1. Obtains the chief complaint (like he did in the problem focused and expanded problem focused histories);
2. Takes an extended history on the present illness or problem;

3. Completes a problem-pertinent system review which includes a review of a limited number of additional systems;
4. Acquires a pertinent *past, family* and/or *social history* directly related to the patients' problems.

Effective in the 1995 **CPT** book, the AMA defined what it meant by "past history" and "social history."

The major difference between the two lower levels of history (problem focused and expanded problem focused) and the detailed one is with the requirement that in a detailed history the physician obtains information about the patient's past history, the patient's family history AND/OR the patient's social history. None of these kinds of histories were required as part of the problem focused and expanded problem focused histories.

In a past patient history, the physician or nurse may ask questions pertaining to any major illnesses or injuries the patient may have had, prior surgeries or hospitalizations (and the reasons behind them), any medications the patient may be taking, whether or not the patient is allergic to anything and, depending on the age of the patient, questions regarding the patient's diet and/or immunizations may also be posed.

The social history may include questions on the patient's marital status (or living arrangements), patient's job or lack of employment, use of drugs, alcohol, tobacco, sexual history, level of education, as well as any other factors that may help the physician more precisely diagnose and/or treat the patient.

For children, social history may include school activities or play activities and interests, questions on socialization, such as what the child is doing and reading, kinds of play, interests in kinds of food, how he or she are getting along in daycare or at school, sleep patterns, etc.

Obtaining the patient's family history could include getting information on the medical events that have taken place in the patient's life or the lives of family members. These could include getting information on the health status/cause of death/diseases of the patient's parents, siblings and children, and any other specific diseases which may relate to why the patient has come for the visit.

An example of a detailed history may be from a patient with recurrent lower back pain (e.g., musculoskeletal system) that radiates to the leg (e.g., neurologic system) or a patient with progressive scoliosis. Notice that the conditions (e.g., recurrent lower back pain or progressive scoliosis) are more complicated than the examples we have discussed thus far. In a detailed history, you will see that more information and background of the patient and the problem is required in order to make a definitive diagnosis.

In the first case (that of the lower back pain), in addition to getting the information that you would in the lower levels of history, the physician must explore events in the patient's past that may have contributed to his current complaint. For example, she might ask the patient what he does for a living and whether he has been doing anything at work that might have caused him to strain his back. In the second case (that of the progressive scoliosis), the physician explores the patient's family history, perhaps asking her if anyone in her family has ever been diagnosed with curvature of the spine, or if any other treatments have been given for the condition.

Comprehensive History

During a comprehensive history, the physician performs the following:

1. Obtains the chief complaint (like he did in the problem-focused, expanded problem-focused and detailed histories);
2. Takes an extended history on the present illness or problem(s);
3. Reviews the systems directly related to the problem or problems as well as all additional body systems;
4. Acquires a complete past family *and* social history.

Notice that the major difference between the comprehensive history and the detailed one is that in the comprehensive history, the patient receives a past patient history AND a past social history AND a past family history. These three types of histories must be included in order for the service to qualify as a comprehensive history.

As an example of the comprehensive history, consider the initial visit of a 73 year-old man with an unexplained 20-pound weight loss. We would ask about the gastrointestinal system and hematologic/lymphatic and immunological systems as well as pose questions about the heart (cardiovascular system) and lungs (respiratory system), review details concerning the eyes, ears, nose and throat, etc.

We would also want to know about any family information (e.g., history of cancer in the family or diabetes), as well as the health status of any siblings and/or children and any other diseases related to the reason(s) the patient was there. In addition to this, we would also obtain information on the patient's use of drugs, alcohol and tobacco, his level of education, his sexual history and preference, his current employment, hobbies or retirement status, his marital status, and any other relevant factors.

In Conclusion

Regardless of the level of detailed information you choose to obtain in your discussions with the patient, you can see that a "history" is a *major ingredient* in determining the appropriate diagnosis of a particular patient on a particular visit. It is for this reason that the history is considered a "key component" of the visit.

The more "intricate" the causes of the patient's complaint are - (e.g., the more difficult it is to "figure out what the diagnosis(es) is(are)"– and the more information required from the patient in order to do so, the higher the "level" of history you will select.

EXAMINATIONS

You will see from the following discussion of examinations, that the names of the levels of examinations are the same as the names for the levels of histories that we just discussed.

Four kinds of examinations are described in **CPT**:

- Problem-Focused Examination
- Expanded Problem-Focused Examination
- Detailed Examination
- Comprehensive Examination

To increase your understanding of these terms, let's explore each of them separately.

Problem-Focused Examination

A problem-focused examination is one that is limited to the affected body area or organ system.

Remember that for the purpose of clarification, body areas are defined as:

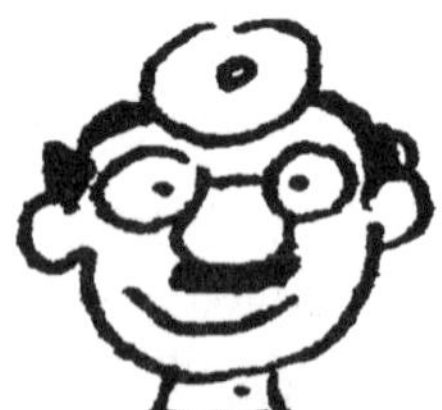

1. Head, which includes the face
2. Neck
3. Chest, breasts and axilla (arm pits)

4. Abdomen
5. Genitalia, groin and buttocks
6. Back
7. Extremities (arms and legs)

Organ systems are, once again:

1. Eyes
2. Ears, nose, mouth and throat
3. Cardiovascular (heart and blood vessels)
4. Respiratory (how you breathe)
5. Gastrointestinal (stomach, intestines, etc.)
6. Genitourinary (genitalia and urinary)
7. Musculoskeletal (muscles and bones)
8. Skin (integumentary)
9. Neurologic (nervous system)
10. Psychiatric
11. Hematologic/lymphatic/immunologic

If you take the definition of "problem-focused" as it applies to exams and you review the systems and body areas listed above, you can see that in a problem focused exam, one affected body area or organ system is examined. For example, a problem-focused exam is the kind your physician would perform on a patient undergoing orthodontics treatment who complains of a wire which is irritating his/her cheek and asks you to check it, or on a patient who had been in the day before to get a blood draw, developed a big bruise or hematoma and needs you to check it. In both cases, notice that the physician is concerned only with the problem at hand and one body area or organ system, and not with anything else that may be affecting the patient.

Expanded Problem-Focused Examination

You will note that, as the name implies, the expanded problem-focused exam is amplified or broadened to encompass more than what was included in the problem focused exam.

In an expanded problem-focused examination, the physician:

1. Examines the affected body organ or system
2. Checks other symptomatic or related organ systems

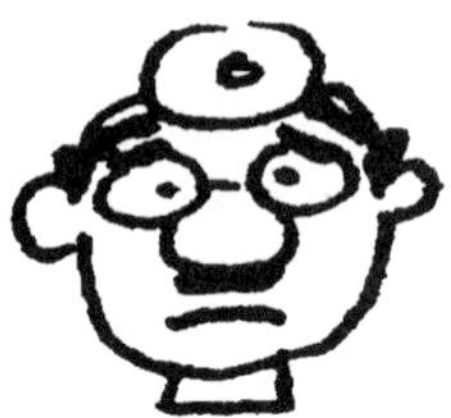

This kind of examination would be performed by a physician on a patient with gradual hearing loss [the physician would check the bones in and around the ears, the eardrums, and related organ systems (e.g., neurologic)] or on a patient with severe acne (the physician would check the face, neck, and probably the back even though the acne may not be found there).

In both of these examples, notice that the physician not only looks at the immediate problem but also examines other problems through systems that may impact the problem at hand. He "expands" the examination.

Detailed Examination

With a detailed examination, the physician performs a more extensive analysis than with a problem-focused or expanded problem-focused examination. During this encounter, the physician performs an extended examination of the affected body area(s) and other symptomatic or related organs. In other words, the patient may come in complaining of one problem which could be connected to or complicated by something else. A physician might conduct a detailed exam on a patient who comes in complaining of flu-like symptoms, nasal discharge and painful teeth/gums. The exam might show an infection in the upper respiratory tract as well as an ear infection and sinus infection. Note that as the definition of detailed exam above describes, you have investigated the affected body area(s) (upper respiratory tract) and the other symptomatic or related organs (e.g., sinuses, ears, throat, nose). With a detailed examination, the physician is concerned about learning as many details as possible.

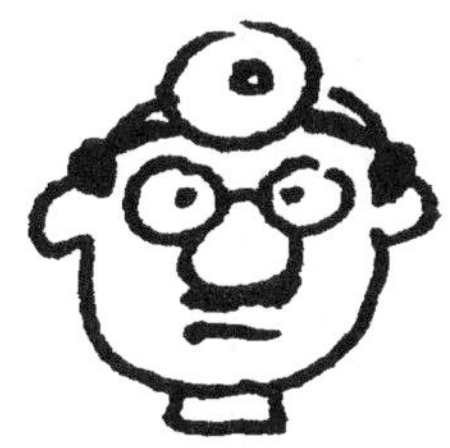

Another example of a detailed examination would be one performed on a patient with recurrent low back pain radiating to the leg. Obviously, the physician would want to get as many details as possible about the patient's back and leg as well as try to find out why the pain is "recurrent." Notice that in this case, the lower back pain impacts the leg and therefore increases the exam from an expanded problem-focused examination to a detailed one by bringing more "systems" into play (e.g., musculoskeletal, neurologic, dermatologic).

You may be thinking that there is only minimal difference between the expanded problem focused exam and the detailed one. At first blush, this seems true. After all, they both cover exams of the affected body area or system and other symptomatic or related organ systems. Upon a closer look, you will see that the difference between the expanded problem-focused exam and the detailed one is the depth of the exam performed. For instance, in the detailed exam, the physician is concerned about obtaining as much information about the related symptomatic organs (those organs may also have "symptoms", or those other organs which the patient complains about) or areas that he or she can. This is because knowing about these others body areas or systems may impact the diagnosis rendered. This in-depth kind of exam is not necessarily required as part of the expanded problem-focused exam which requires perhaps a look or two but which may or may not impact the overall diagnosis if an extensive exam is not made.

In the case described above, it was evident that when the person complained of lower back pain that radiated out to the leg that his condition could have been caused by several different reasons (e.g., pinched nerve, prior injury) and, the problem could impact the function of other body parts (e.g., the movement of the lower leg, problems with the rotation of the ankle or knee). When you understand that reviewing and examining other body parts and their relationships to the patient's main complaint can sometimes only be accomplished through an in-depth examination such as you find as part of the detailed visit, it is helpful to know that this kind of examination is here for your use.

Comprehensive Examination

Here the physician performs a complete single system specialty examination or a complete multisystem examination.

The **American Heritage Dictionary** defines complete as:

> ***complete:*** *"having all necessary or normal parts."*

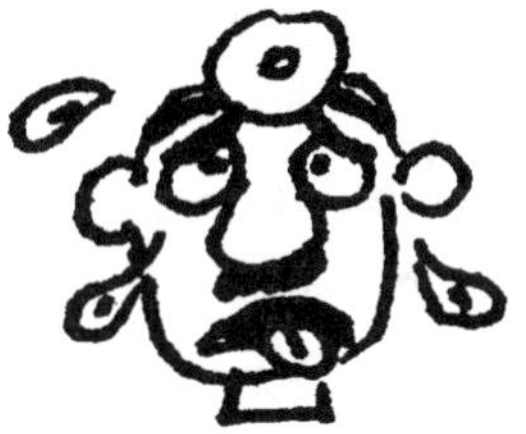

During this kind of examination, the physician must be sure that every part of the system is explored or that each necessary component of a group of systems is investigated.

Your physician would likely perform a comprehensive examination on a patient with systemic vasculitis (inflammation of the blood vessels) that has caused decreased circulation to the legs. Note that the blood vessels travel all over the body and vasculitis (inflammation of the vessels) could occur anywhere in the body, thereby necessitating that the physician check many systems and body areas. Another example where a comprehensive exam would be performed would be on a patient with severe persistent obstructive lung disease, congestive heart failure, and hypertension. In both of these examples (the systemic vasculitis and the severe persistent obstructive lung disease), the physician looks at all systems involved. In the first case, it may be the circulatory and musculoskeletal systems; in the second case, it may be the circulatory, respiratory, and renal systems.

Keep in mind that the comprehensive examination may involve more than one system and always includes performing an exhaustive check. Also keep in mind that many physicians like to code for "comprehensive" exams because they claim that they always provide a thorough physical. It is very important **NOT** to confuse a comprehensive type exam as described by the **CPT** book and the word "comprehensive" (AKA a thorough exam) terminology used by the physician. These "comprehensive" services would be very different; that is, you could provide a very thorough exam on a single system in one area (e.g., the ears) but still not qualify in a comprehensive exam in terms of the **CPT** definition for comprehensive.

Now that we have discussed the four kinds of histories and the four kinds of examinations, let's move on to the kinds of medical decisions the physician can make.

Medical Decision-Making

As was just discussed, the kind of history and exam you choose *are only two* of the "key" ingredients in selecting a particular type of evaluation and management service. Many physicians and/or coders make the big mistake of basing the "level of service" they pick for and evaluation and management code (e.g., 99201 through 99205) upon how "thorough" they think they were in providing an evaluation and management-type service to a patient. In other words, they only take into account the history and exam and do not stop to analyze the other key ingredient (i.e., medical decision-making) that is extremely important in making an overall selection of a code. This is not the thing to do! As an example, I have seen many physicians say that since they completely and thoroughly checked a patient's knee and even took x-rays they should be able to code for a comprehensive level of service. This is not necessarily true. As you will learn, making a decision about the level you choose to describe what was done for a patient in evaluation and management services is dependent upon *all* key components as they apply to a new or an established patient. Let us review the four kinds of medical decision-making in order to be able to put the entire picture together as to what components are necessary in accurately selecting a level of evaluation and management service.

Kinds of Medical Decision Making

Four basic kinds of medical decision-making are defined in **CPT**:

- Straightforward
- Low Complexity
- Moderate Complexity
- High Complexity

According to the AMA, medical decision-making refers to the difficulty a physician has in establishing a diagnosis for the patient and/or in deciding what next to do for the patient. For example, should she treat him? Should she run more tests? The degree of difficulty involved will vary from case to case because some conditions are more difficult to diagnose than others, and one treatment may be better for some patients than for others with the same diagnosis. For this reason, the AMA has specified three elements that need to be considered in selecting the kind of decision-making that is rendered by the physician.

These elements are:

1. The number of diagnoses or management options available to the physician (i.e., Does he or she have a lot or just a little to consider here?);

2. The amount and/or complexity of data to be reviewed (Is the patient having a variety of tests that will need to be evaluated? Has the patient or another physician sent in data that needs to be reviewed?); and

3. The risk of complications and/or other serious injury or illness (morbidity) or death (mortality) of the patient (Is there a chance that the patient will get sicker or even die if not treated immediately or in a certain way? Do more tests need to be run to further narrow down the possibilities? Is there enough time to run these tests?).

By looking at the chart, you will see that going across the page is listed the kinds of decision making that can be made (i.e., straightforward, low, moderate or high). Going down the page, the "y" axis", you can see the different elements that need to be considered in order to make a final selection of the kind of decision (i.e., number of diagnosis or management options, amount of data to check and the risk of complications). In order to effectively select the correct kind of medical decision making made, all three of the items found on the "y" axis need to be considered individually.

CHART A KIND OF DECISION-MAKING				
Element	**Straight-Forward**	**Low**	**Moderate**	**High**
Number of diagnoses	Minimal	Limited	Multiple	Extensive
Amount of data to check	Minimal or none	Limited	Moderate	Extensive
Risk of more serious illness or death	Minimal	Low	Moderate	High

For example, let's say your physician saw a patient with one diagnosis, with very little data to be checked, and with a minimal risk of more serious illness or death to the patient. Going to the chart, you would mark each of these items by matching up as closely as possible the one diagnosis with the word that it most closely resembles (e.g., minimal). Likewise, the small amount of data to check could be matched against the word that mostly closely describes this (minimal) and the low risk of morbidity or mortality could be matched up to what it most closely resembles (minimal). If you were to circle each of these terms on the chart, your chart would look like the one labeled as Chart A.

The rules in **CPT** say that two of the three "words" that correspond to each element (e.g., minimal, limited, moderate) must be equal or exceeded. For example, in order to qualify for a straightforward decision, the word "minimal" must be circled (on the chart), at least two out of the three times. See Chart A.

Think of this as you would when you learned about fractions. Remember when your teacher would ask you to look at the highest "common denominator?" Picking out the *kind* of medical decision-making made is similar to that. You need to look for what word appears the most often or, stated in another way, what word have you at least met (or exceeded) three of the three times.

To illustrate this, take a look at the following lineal drawing. On it you will see the kind of medical decision making. By charting the words minimal, limited/low, multiple/moderate, or extensive/high next to the # of diagnosis, amount of data to review and risk of complications and or morbidity or mortality, you can see which word (i.e., minimal, limited, multiple or extensive) you met or exceeded two of the three times. As you can see, at least for this first example, the word you met or exceeded in three of the three cases was minimal.

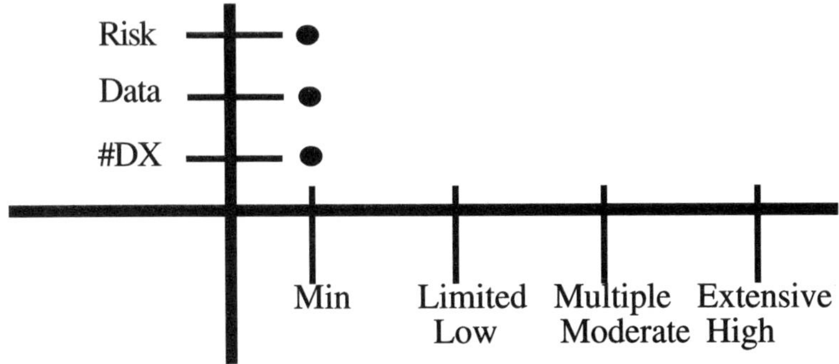

In considering another example, let's say your physician saw someone who had two diagnoses (see the word limited circled on Chart B for number of diagnoses), a limited amount of data to be checked (see the word limited circled on Chart B for amount of data to check), and minimal risk of complications (see the word minimal circled on Chart B for risk of more serious death or illness). From the chart, you can see that your physician has met two elements needed for the low complexity decision-making level and has not met that level in the risk of complications category. The rules say that **two of three** elements must be met or exceeded in order to qualify for a particular decision-making level.

CHART B KIND OF DECISION-MAKING				
Element	**Straight-Forward**	**Low**	**Moderate**	**High**
Number of diagnoses	Minimal	Limited	Multiple	Extensive
Amount of data to check	Minimal or none	Limited	Moderate	Extensive
Risk of more serious illness or death	Minimal	Low	Moderate	High

Your physician has met the two thirds criteria for the low complexity medical decision-making. You would select low complexity decision-making.

Another example would be if the patient had an extensive number of diagnoses [e.g., hypertension, epilepsy, dementia, Alzheimers, old age, mental retardation - (see the word extensive circled on Chart C for number of diagnoses), a moderate amount of data to check multiple lab results, blood tests, EKGs, X-rays, etc. (see the word moderate circled on Chart C for amount of data to check) and a low risk of dying due to any "treatment" that was prescribed (see the word low circled on Chart C for the risk of serious illness or death).] In this case, the decision-making would be considered moderate (see Chart C) based on the two out of three rule as described earlier in this chapter. Continue to play with these charts until you get the hang of it and truly feel comfortable with the two out of the three rule.

CHART C
KIND OF DECISION-MAKING

Element	**Straight-Forward**	**Low**	**Moderate**	**High**
Number of diagnoses	Minimal	Limited	Multiple	Extensive
Amount of data to check	Minimal or none	Limited	Moderate	Extensive
Risk of more serious illness or death	Minimal	Low	Moderate	High

Note that in order to accurately code, each of the key ingredients of the Evaluation and Management service must be taken into account.

TIME

In the Evaluation and Management Section, time is defined in two ways:

- Face-to-face time
- Unit/floor time

Face-to-Face Time

Face-to-face time is time the physician spends examining the patient, taking a history, and talking with the patient. It is, as its name implies, time spent with the patient and/or family. Consider the following example:

99201 *Office or other outpatient visit for the Evaluation and Management of a new patient, which requires these three key components:*

- *A problem-focused history;*
- *A problem-focused examination;*
- *Straightforward medical decision-making*

Counseling and/or coordination of care with other providers or agencies are provided consistent with the nature of the problem(s) and the patient's and/or family's needs.

Usually, the presenting problem(s) are self-limited or minor. Physicians typically spend 10 minutes face-to-face with the patient and/or family.

Notice that the amount of time listed is 10 minutes. This is an average length of time for this kind of visit. Some visits may take a little longer, and others may not take as long. Some physicians may take more time and others less.

These 10 minutes are spent **with the patient and/or family**. They do not include the time the staff spent to make the appointment. Nor do they include the time the physician spent reviewing records and lab reports or speaking with other health care professionals involved in caring for the patient, such as hospital staff, nursing home staff, and therapists. All of this time spent on behalf of the patient when the patient is not present is called non-face-to-face time.

Non-face-to-face time is not included in the amount of time listed with codes for office visits and consultations. It is, however, included within the relative value figure calculated for total "work" involved in providing the service. Thus, non-face-to-face time is reflected in the *payment* for E/M services provided to a Medicare patient.

Unit/Floor Time

Unit/floor time is time the physician spends on the patient's unit or floor (inpatient hospital surgery unit, OB/GYN floor) reading or establishing the patient's chart, examining the patient at his or her bedside, jotting down notes about the patient's progress, ordering tests, communicating with nurses and other staff, and counseling the patient and/or the patient's family.

There may also be time in which the physician is not on the floor. This is not included in the **CPT** definition of unit/floor time. For example, the physician may be in the radiology department reviewing x-rays. This off-floor time *was* considered in determining Medicare's relative value units for inpatient Evaluation and Management services.

As you might expect, unit/floor time is used with services provided to patients who are bedridden and admitted to a facility.

The Role of Time in Coding

Normally, the amount of time spent either face-to-face with the patient or on the patient's unit/floor is not a deciding factor when choosing an Evaluation and Management code.

In certain cases, however, the amount of face-to-face or on floor/unit time **does** become the deciding factor. Time can take precedence over those key components (history, examination, and medical decision-making) that normally are the deciding factors for the kind of visit chosen. If the time spent counseling the patient on issues directly related to the presenting problem or coordinating patient care becomes greater than 50% of the total time for the visit, time becomes the deciding factor.

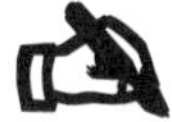

Please note that TIME ONLY becomes the deciding factor in determining the correct E & M code when more than 50% of the face-to-face or on unit/floor time is spent on counseling or coordination of care.

For example, let's say an established patient with stable cirrhosis of the liver comes in for a normal visit. The physician performs an expanded problem-focused history and expanded problem-focused examination, and makes a straightforward medical decision, all of which takes about 10 minutes. Following the history examination and medical decision, the patient begins to explain to the physician that she and her husband aren't getting along and that she has started drinking again. The physician spends an additional 15 minutes counseling the patient on how these activities can impact her condition. What was a 10-minute history and exam has become a 25-minute visit. In this case, time is the deciding coding factor, since counseling was more than 50% of the face-to-face time.

The scale below illustrates this example.

5 Minutes	3 Minutes	2 Minutes	15 Minutes
History	Exam	Medical Decision	Counseling

Total Visit 25 Minutes

As you can see, the counseling portion (15 minutes) took more than the time that it took to do the history and exam (total history/exam time = 10 minutes; 15 minutes of counseling > 10 minutes of history and exam time).

Since the visit (without the counseling) would have been an expanded problem-focused visit (99213) before the counseling, and since the time spent in counseling was greater than 50% of the time it took to do the history, exam, and medical decision, you would choose the Evaluation and Management code with a 25-minute time frame. In this example, you would choose code 99214.

As you can see, the use of these Evaluation and Management codes must be precise. It is critical that you understand all of the parameters with which you must work.

PUTTING IT ALL TOGETHER

The greatest problem that a coder faces is to accurately code the E/M section. The reason that it is difficult is because it requires a judgment on the part of the coder or physician.

It is of critical importance to note that not all of your encounters with patients will fit neatly into the prepackaged descriptions listed in the **CPT** book. You won't always have, for example, a problem-focused history, problem-focused exam and straight-forward medical-mecisions as described in the 99201 code.

You will see that you may provide a problem-focused history on a person and an expanded problem-focused exam, and there would be no exact code description given in **CPT** to describe this scenario. Because of this, let's talk about an easy way to implement these ideas in a manner that will help you select accurate visit codes for all patient/physician encounters. You can do this by using the following form, called the **DOC** Form. The **DOC** stands for "Doctor's Office Checklist."

The DOC form allows the physician to easily take an active part in the E/M coding decision, and allows the coder to work with greater speed (rather than having to constantly ask the doctor - what exactly did you do, what body parts did you examine, what kind of decision did you make, what was/were the diagnosis (es) how long did it take you to reach your decision, and so on).

There are two sides to the actual form. One side describes services that occur in the office/outpatient setting. These include:

1. Office/outpatient visits (for both new and established patients);

and

2. Consultations (including both outpatient and confirmatory consultations).

DOC FORM

	OFFICE/OUTPATIENT		CONSULTATION	
	New(3)	Established(2)	Office/O.P.(3)	Confirm(3)
Minimal service		99211		
HISTORY				
Problem-Focused	99201	99212	99241	99271
Exp/Prob-Focused	99202	99213	99242	99272
Detailed	99203	99214	99243	99273
Comprehensive	99204/5	99215	99244/5	99274/5
EXAMINATION				
Problem-Focused	99201	99212	99241	99271
Exp/Prob-Focused	99202	99213	99242	99272
Detailed	99203	99214	99243	99273
Comprehensive	99204/5	99215	99244/5	99274/5
MEDICAL DECISION MAKING				
Straight-Forward	99201/2	99212	99241/2	99271/2
Low Complexity	99203	99213	99243	99273
Mod Complexity	99204	99214	99244	99274
High Complexity	99205	99215	99245	99275
TIME: Total ______		Counsel/Coord. of Care: ______		
10 minutes	99201	99212		
15		99213	99241	
20	99202			
25		99214		
30	99203		99242	
40		99215	99243	
45	99204			
60	99205		99244	
80			99245	

Patient Name:______________________________

Date: ____________ Physician's Signature:______________________

MedBooks 101 West Buckingham, Richardson, Texas 75081
1-800-443-7397

The other side of the DOC form includes Evaluation and Management services that occur in the hospital setting. These included:

1. Consultations (including in patient, follow-up and confirmatory consultations);

2. Emergency services (for both new and established patients)

   and,

3. Hospital inpatient visits (for both an initial and subsequent visits).

Let's begin our study of the DOC from by looking at the first side, the office/outpatient side.

As you scan the DOC form (from left to right), you can see that both Office/Outpatient Visits and Consultations are listed at the top. As was previously stated, these two kinds of services have been placed together on this particular DOC form because both are rendered in the office/outpatient setting.

Beneath each of these services is a further explanation of the encounter. For example, the words "New (3)" and "Established (2)" under the bold heading of **Office/Outpatient Visits** tell whether the patient is new to the physician or established. Additionally, it tells us that either three (see the parenthesis next to the word "new") or two (see the parenthesis next to the word "established") key components will be required to code and bill for these services. In the exact same way, the words "Office/ Outpatient" with the parenthesis and the number 3, and the word "Confirmatory" with the parenthesis and the number 3 under the bold heading of **Consultations** tell us about these services, explaining different kinds of consultations and how many key components are required in order to code for each.

DOC FORM

	OFFICE/OUTPATIENT		CONSULTATION	
	New(3)	Established(2)	Office/O.P.(3)	Confirm(3)
Minimal service		99211		
HISTORY				
Problem-Focused	99201	99212	99241	99271
Exp/Prob-Focused	99202	99213	99242	99272
Detailed	99203	99214	99243	99273
Comprehensive	99204/5	99215	99244/5	99274/5
EXAMINATION				
Problem-Focused	99201	99212	99241	99271

Going from the top of the page to the bottom, you can see that the key components of the visits (e.g., history, exam, and medical decision-making).

Although time is not considered a key component, it does influence the code selected when the portion of the visit concerning counseling or coordination of care takes more than 50% of the total encounter.

When you look at the DOC form, you will see that time is listed at the bottom following the three key components.

As you can see by looking at the form, a space follows the word "time". In this space, your physician should mark the amount of time spent with the patient. In most circumstances, the number

High Complexity	99205	99215	99245	99275
TIME: Total ________	Counsel/Coord. of Care: ________			
10 minutes	99201	99212		
15		99213	99241	
20	99202			
25		99214		
30	99203		99242	
40		99215	99243	
45	99204			
60	99205		99244	
80			99245	

Patient Name:________________________

Date: ____________ Physician's Signature:________________

MedBooks 101 West Buckingham, Richardson, Texas 75081
1-800-443-7397

WARNING: This product is copyrighted and is not to be duplicated in any manner without express written permission from MedBooks.

www.medbooks.com

of minutes will be consistent with the average length of time listed for the service in the code description. Your physician can also circle the amount of time spent as it is listed under the **Time** heading. Listing the amount of time on the form is a good habit, even if counseling or coordination of care is not the dominant factor controlling the visit. If you consistently list it, you can be sure it will be there when you need it.

Using The DOC Form In The Office/Outpatient Environment

Let's do an exercise to show how you can piece this whole thing together. Suppose a 10 year-old new patient comes into your office complaining of itching on his leg. Your physician takes a problem-focused history (records the patient's name and age, finds out how he got the rash, determines whether he has any allergies) and completes a problem-focused examination (looks at the rash, notices how red it is, notices if it is inflamed). Your physician decides that the patient has poison oak and that he needs a certain lotion (straightforward decision-making). The physician writes down the name of the lotion for the patient, tells him how to use it, and thanks him for coming in. The entire visit takes about 10 minutes.

As you look at the DOC form, you will circle the following:

- Problem-Focused History
- Problem-Focused Examination
- Straightforward Medical Decision-Making

You will also indicate 10 minutes in the space provided for the total time.

Example 6.1

DOC FORM

	OFFICE/OUTPATIENT		CONSULTATION	
	New(3)	Established(2)	Office/O.P.(3)	Confirm(3)
Minimal service		99211		
HISTORY				
Problem-Focused	(99201)	99212	99241	99271
Exp/Prob-Focused	99202	99213	99242	99272
Detailed	99203	99214	99243	99273
Comprehensive	99204/5	99215	99244/5	99274/5
EXAMINATION				
Problem-Focused	(99201)	99212	99241	99271
Exp/Prob-Focused	99202	99213	99242	99272
Detailed	99203	99214	99243	99273
Comprehensive	99204/5	99215	99244/5	99274/5
MEDICAL DECISION-MAKING				
Straight-Forward	(99201/2)	99212	99241/2	99271/2
Low Complexity	99203	99213	99243	99273
Mod Complexity	99204	99214	99244	99274
High Complexity	99205	99215	99245	99275
TIME: Total 10		Counsel/Coord. of Care:		
10 minutes	99201	99212		
15		99213	99241	
20	99202			
25		99214		
30	99203		99242	
40		99215	99243	
45	99204			
60	99205		99244	
80			99245	

Patient Name:__________

Date: ________ Physician's Signature:__________

MedBooks 101 West Buckingham, Richardson, Texas 75081

1-800-443-7397

www.medbooks.com

As you can see from the DOC Form, under **New Patient**, you should choose the 99201 code because you circled 99201 at least three times (see Example 6.1). This means your physician met or exceeded the required number in at least three cases. The reason this number must be met (indicated by the same code number) or exceeded (indicated by a greater number) in at least three cases is that three key components are required for this visit. You were reminded that you needed three key components when you saw "New (3)" under Office/Outpatient Visits.

On a lineal scale this example would appear as follows:

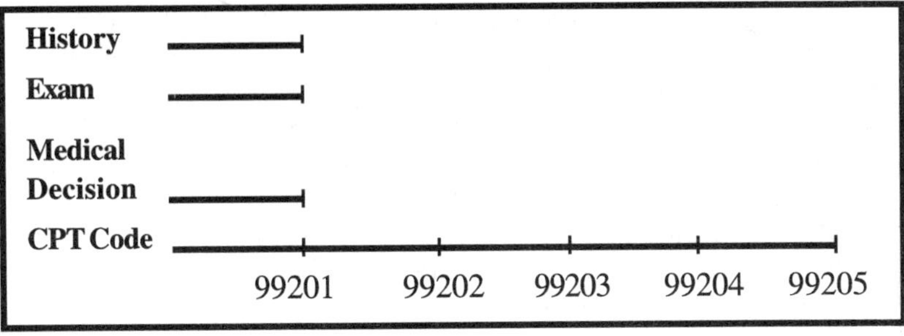

Notice that you met the number 99201 three out of the three required times for this new patient.

Let's take another example (see Example 6.2). Suppose a second new patient comes into your office with the same complaint (poison oak). This time, your physician provides exactly the same services she provided for the first patient

Example 6.2

DOC FORM

	OFFICE/OUTPATIENT		CONSULTATION	
	New(3)	Established(2)	Office/O.P.(3)	Confirm(3)
Minimal service		99211		
HISTORY				
Problem-Focused	(99201)	99212	99241	99271
Exp/Prob-Focused	99202	99213	99242	99272
Detailed	99203	99214	99243	99273
Comprehensive	99204/5	99215	99244/5	99274/5
EXAMINATION				
Problem-Focused	(99201)	99212	99241	99271
Exp/Prob-Focused	99202	99213	99242	99272
Detailed	99203	99214	99243	99273
Comprehensive	99204/5	99215	99244/5	99274/5
MEDICAL DECISION-MAKING				
Straight-Forward	(99201/2)	99212	99241/2	99271/2
Low Complexity	99203	99213	99243	99273
Mod Complexity	99204	99214	99244	99274
High Complexity	99205	99215	99245	99275
TIME: Total	30	Counsel/Coord. of Care:		
10 minutes	99201	99212		
15		99213	99241	
20	99202			
25		99214		
30	(99203)		99242	
40		99215	99243	
45	99204			
60	99205		99244	
80			99245	

Patient Name:________________

Date: ________ Physician's Signature:________________

MedBooks 101 West Buckingham, Richardson, Texas 75081

1-800-443-7397

www.medbooks.com

(problem-focused history and examination with straightforward decision-making). At the end of the visit, however, the mother of this boy goes on to explain that her son has had problems concentrating in school and asks for some advice on what to do. In other words, this "10-minute visit" has taken 30 minutes!

By looking at the circles on your DOC Form, you can see that the correct code to use is 99203 because the additional time was spent in counseling.

The reason 99203 is the correct code for the second example is that the counseling was greater than 50% of the total time. Notice that the code associated with the 30-minute time frame was the code 99203.

Let's take one final example. Suppose an established patient who seems very ill comes into the office. Your physician performs an expanded problem-focused history and an expanded problem-focused examination. Because of the number of management options he has to consider, the amount and complexity of the data he has to review, and the risk of complications associated with various treatments, your physician makes a treatment decision that is moderately complex. The DOC form (see Example 6.3) illustrates this.

As you can see, the circled codes are 99213 for the history, 99213 for the examination, and 99214 for the decision-making. Because this is an established patient, two key components must be met or exceeded to qualify for the visit (see Example 6.3)

Example 6.3

DOC FORM

	OFFICE/OUTPATIENT		CONSULTATION	
	New(3)	Established(2)	Office/O.P.(3)	Confirm(3)
Minimal service		99211		
HISTORY				
Problem-Focused	99201	99212	99241	99271
Exp/Prob-Focused	99202	(99213)	99242	99272
Detailed	99203	99214	99243	99273
Comprehensive	99204/5	99215	99244/5	99274/5
EXAMINATION				
Problem-Focused	99201	99212	99241	99271
Exp/Prob-Focused	99202	(99213)	99242	99272
Detailed	99203	99214	99243	99273
Comprehensive	99204/5	99215	99244/5	99274/5
MEDICAL DECISION-MAKING				
Straight-Forward	99201/2	99212	99241/2	99271/2
Low Complexity	99203	99213	99243	99273
Mod Complexity	99204	(99214)	99244	99274
High Complexity	99205	99215	99245	99275
TIME: Total ________		Counsel/Coord. of Care:		________
10 minutes	99201	99212		
15		99213	99241	
20	99202			
25		99214		
30	99203		99242	
40		99215	99243	
45	99204			
60	99205		99244	
80			99245	

Patient Name:____________________

Date: ____________ Physician's Signature:____________________

MedBooks 101 West Buckingham, Richardson, Texas 75081

1-800-443-7397

www.medbooks.com

Looking at this on the lineal scale you can see that 99213 has been met twice and exceeded once (by 99214). Because 99213 has been exceeded only once (and **two** key components have to be met or exceeded), you must choose 99213.

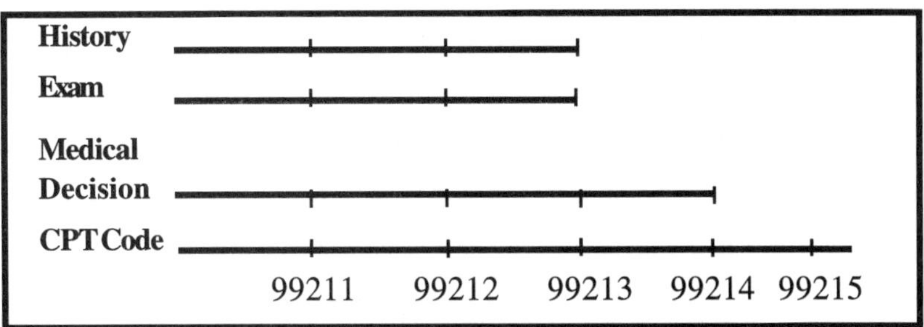

There are many systems available for choosing the appropriate E/M code. The DOC form is only one of them. Check with your supplier for either the DOC Form or another system.

On a final note, many people will tell you that it is better for you (if you can) to code and bill for a new patient visit because it pays more. This is not necessarily true. Because of the three-out-of-three rule for new patients and two-out-of-three rule for established ones, you may find that the exact same kind of visit may render two very different levels of service.

To illustrate this, let's say you saw a normal, healthy, 24-year old patient for her yearly physical. If she were a new patient and your decision-making were straightforward – even though you may have done a head to toe check with a pap smear and obtained a comprehensive history – you would need to code that visit as a 99202 or 99203. This would be because of the fact that three of the three key components (i.e., history, exam and medical decision making) must be met, and the medical decision-making portion brought you down to a straightforward or low complexity level (see DOC form). This same patient on an established level might be coded as a 99215 because only two of the three key components are required – which you qualify for under your history and exam (i.e., you met the 99215 under history and 99215 under exam because both of them are comprehensive). See example 6.4 on the following page. It's probably good for you to work this example out using the DOC form tools contained herein. Once you can "see" this example of the DOC form and once you go through the "process" of having to figure out the medical decision-making, all of this will really make sense to you.

Example 6.4

DOC FORM

	OFFICE/OUTPATIENT		CONSULTATION	
	New(3)	Established(2)	Office/O.P.(3)	Confirm(3)
Minimal service		99211		
HISTORY				
Problem-Focused	99201	99212	99241	99271
Exp/Prob-Focused	99202	99213	99242	99272
Detailed	99203	99214	99243	99273
Comprehensive	(99204/5)	(99215)	99244/5	99274/5
EXAMINATION				
Problem-Focused	99201	99212	99241	99271
Exp/Prob-Focused	99202	99213	99242	99272
Detailed	99203	99214	99243	99273
Comprehensive	(99204/5)	(99215)	99244/5	99274/5
MEDICAL DECISION-MAKING				
Straight-Forward	(99201/2)	(99212)	99241/2	99271/2
Low Complexity	99203	99213	99243	99273
Mod Complexity	99204	99214	99244	99274
High Complexity	99205	99215	99245	99275
TIME: Total ________		Counsel/Coord. of Care:		________
10 minutes	99201	99212		
15		99213	99241	
20	99202			
25		99214		
30	99203		99242	
40		99215	99243	
45	99204			
60	99205		99244	
80			99245	

Patient Name:______________________________

Date: ____________ Physician's Signature:______________________

MedBooks 101 West Buckingham, Richardson, Texas 75081

1-800-443-7397

www.medbooks.com

Now let's move on to a discussion of the nuances in each subsection.

Office Or Other Outpatient Services

The Office/Outpatient subsection is divided into two parts: visits for new patients (those who have not received any professional services from the physician in the past three years) and visits for established patients (those who **have** received professional services in the past three years). (See exact definitions of new and established patients at the beginning of this chapter.) Once you have determined whether the patient is new or established, you must determine the degree of history, physical examination, and medical decision-making performed in the visit.

It is important for you to understand that your "office" may be located in a stand-alone facility or in a hospital. **Where** it is located doesn't matter. As long as it's your office, you qualify to use these office-visit codes.

An outpatient facility is one where the patient may be seen before being admitted to a hospital, nursing facility, or observation unit. These sites may include your office or some other ambulatory facility. If your physician is seeing patients in these environments, you can appropriately code for histories, examinations, and medical decisions rendered by using the Office/ Outpatient Evaluation and Management codes.

If during the course of the patient encounter, your physician decides that the patient needs to be admitted to a hospital or nursing facility, you will have to use the codes from one of those sections and **not** the Office/Outpatient codes. Likewise, if your physician decides that the patient needs to be observed and followed until a decision to admit the patient is made, you would use the Hospital Observation service codes.

As you can see by looking at the Evaluation and Management codes described earlier, each time frame listed is the average length of time a particular visit takes among many different specialties. Don't get hung up on these time frames. What we said before bears repeating: An Evaluation and Management service deals with what the physician does during the time he or she spends with the patient, **not** with the amount of time itself. The exception is when the physician spends more than 50% of the total time in counseling and coordination of care.

As we also said earlier, remembering that time is not a "key ingredient" is one of the best things you can do for your office. Many billers cause a considerable loss of time and money for their physicians by not paying attention to the definitions and uses of key components. Insurance carriers have had many problems in the past with physicians who misused the "levels of service" in prior versions of **CPT**. As a result, implementation and use of the Evaluation and Management codes is monitored very closely.

Although it is not a substitute for written documentation, use of the DOC form (in conjunction with patient progress notes) may protect the practice in an insurance audit. With the DOC form and your physician's complete notes in the medical record, you can easily show how you've followed the rules for **CPT** Evaluation and Management codes in your billing practices.

Many a coder has made the grim mistake of choosing codes for one of the following reasons:

1. We need to code it that way to get the money our office requires for this type of examination.

2. The Evaluation and Management codes just don't pay correctly.

Using either of these reasons can cause your office trouble if you are audited by an insurance carrier.

Medicare (like the IRS) has the authority to audit each and every physician's office for misuse of codes. If a physician's office is found in violation of the coding rules, that physician may be required to repay all overcharges to the Medicare program or even be barred from participating in the program.

Medicare carriers can often tell by their internal computers which codes your office uses most often. They track the charges submitted by your office and the codes you have used to submit those charges. For example, if your office only uses the Evaluation and Management code that describes a comprehensive history and examination (99204) for every new patient, the carrier's computer will show only this number on your office's history of charges for new patients.

Keep in mind that to carriers, not all patients fall into the same category. The old days of charging all new patients the same fee for the first visit, regardless of what the physician does, are gone. You must now code each patient visit according to the specific levels of judgment exercised by your physician during the visits.

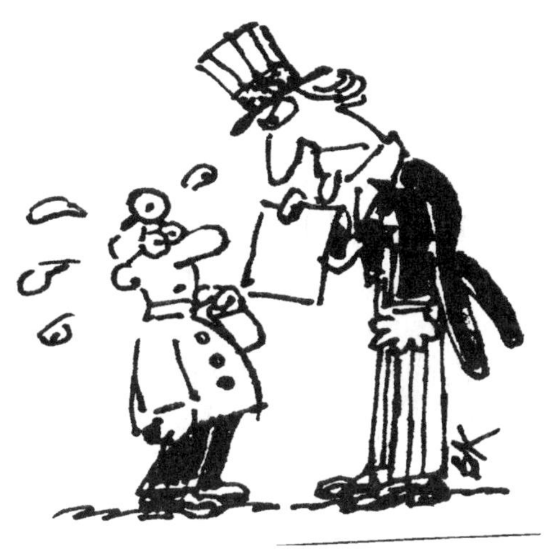

Medicare, like the IRS, has the authority to audit...

The point of coding according to the level of expertise exercised in the patient/physician encounter cannot be overstressed! A little care on the front end could save your office hours of work and headaches on the back end during an audit.

Hospital Observation Services

The Hospital Observation services codes describe the Evaluation and Management services provided to patients in an "observation unit" or in "observation status" at the hospital. These codes are to be used only by the primary or admitting physician. Remember that although these codes describe Evaluation and Management services, they should not be used to describe services rendered to patients following surgery (for example, recovery room services because the concept of the global Surgical Package includes pre-op and post-op and the recovery room portion of the care following surgery would be considered part of the post-op care). Likewise, the Evaluation and Management codes do not describe any other "procedure" that may happen in an observation area (such as the taking of an x-ray, performance of lab tests, or placement of a catheter).

There are some hospitals that do not have an "official" hospital observation area set up for patients. In these facilities, patients may be "observed" in the emergency room, or in some other area that is designated as an observation area for that facility. The important thing here is not necessarily "where" the patient received the observation services as much as it is the *kind* of services (i.e., observation services) that the patient receives.

There are several questions that you may have concerning the Hospital Observation services codes. The first is what code to use if a patient is seen for a second day (new 24-hour period) in the observation unit and not admitted to the hospital or sent home. You will notice that **CPT** only addresses initial observation care and not any "subsequent" visits. Remember, the purpose of "observation" is to see what's going on with the patient. In all likelihood a diagnosis will be established within 24 hours. At the end of 24 hours, the patient will either be admitted to the hospital for further tests and care or discharged. Therefore, if a patient continues to be monitored for a second 24-hour period, you should either ask your doctor if the patient was admitted (and maybe this fact was just not mentioned in the chart or physician's notes) and code for the hospital admission or perhaps the patient seen in "observation" for the second date was also discharged on that date and you could use the Observation Care Discharge service code, 99217. If neither of these codes will work for you, you will need to use an unlisted procedure code (in this case 99499) to indicate that you provided a service that does not have a code.

The second question relates to the suggestion by **CPT** for a physician who sees the patient in the observation unit but who is not the "admitting" physician. **CPT** suggests that the non-admitting physician should use the office or other outpatient "consultation" codes (99241-99245). Although this may be appropriate for a doctor who is rendering his or her opinion about a patient in the observation unit, it is important for the reader to keep in mind that the use of the Office/Outpatient *"consultation"* codes would not be correct for the physician who is in fact treating the patient while in this area. We will talk more about ***why*** it would be incorrect to use the consultation codes for treatment purposes once we get to consultations in the next few pages.

Consider the following example: Suppose a pregnant patient were admitted to the observation unit for the monitoring of premature contractions. At the same time, because of her pregnancy and severe infection in her eye, she is being seen and treated daily by her ophthalmologist. Because her ophthalmologist is treating her (and not rendering his or her opinion), it would not be consistent with the definition of a consultation for the doctor to code the office or other outpatient consultation visits. The physician (in this case, the opthalmologist) who is treating the patient while the other is observing the patient should code his or her services by using the Office or Other Outpatient Services.

There are three additional situations which can be confusing in coding for Hospital Observation services:

a. When someone is admitted to the observation unit and discharged that same day (use only the codes 99234-99236);

b. When the patient is admitted to the observation unit and then not discharged until the next day (use 99218-99220 for the first day and 99217 for the day that they are discharged and sent home);

c. When the patient is admitted to the observation unit and then, on the second day, admitted to the hospital. In this case, code for the hospital observation on the first day and the hospital admission on the second day (see codes 99221-99223).

Let's take some examples. Let's say that a patient has been in a car accident and comes into the ER unconscious via an ambulance at around 11:00 p.m. The ER physician examines the patient and finds that all vitals are in good working order (the heart is beating well, the lungs sound good and clear, the pulse is as it should be), the patient has no broken bones, so the ER doctor decides to admit the patient to observation until the patient "comes to" (gains consciousness). The patient finally comes to on the next "date". You would bill these services using only the Hospital Observation code for the first day since the same physician provided both the ER and the admission to the observation unit and the Observation Discharge service code (99217) for the next "date".

Here is another one. Suppose you are diabetic and are currently being treated by a physician in internal medicine. Over the weekend, you experience severe dizziness. You go to the emergency room where the emergency room physician does a preliminary workup but is unable to locate any specific reasons for your dizziness (e.g., you have no sinus conditions, your physician recently performed an EEG and found no problems and you have been taking your medication as prescribed). Since you have been working with your doctor for years, you ask the ER physician to please have your doctor called and advised of your being at the hospital.

Once the ER physician has spoken to your doctor, he returns and says that your physician wants you admitted to the observation area and that your doctor has given the orders for such an admission to the nurse over the phone. You are wheeled down to Observation where your physician meets with you and goes over the findings of the ER doctor.

To code for this, you must first note that two physicians are providing services here, the ER doctor and your internal medicine physician. You may think at first that you can only code for the higher of the two E/M services for either doctor (i.e., the Hospital Observation code – see 99218-99220) since two Evaluation and Management services occurred on the same date. As the **CPT** book points out, however, this would only be true if the same physician rendered the two E/M services. In our example case, two separate physicians rendered the two E/M services and, therefore, each doctor's service can be coded and billed.

Finally, let's say you go to your physician complaining of a severe headache. Your doctor takes a history consistent with your complaints, examines you and prescribes some special migraine medicine. Since it is almost 5:00 p.m., and since you have no one at home to take care of you, your doctor also decides that it would be best to admit you to the observation unit to make sure that the medication has in fact cleared up this pain in your head. Your doctor does not order any kind of EEG or CAT scan because you have no insurance and have never had any headache of this kind. After about 45 minutes of being in the observation unit, you feel better than you have in years. Your physician discharges you and sends you home. Coding for this example would simply be the code for the Observation or Inpatient

Care Services, 99234-99236, which include the observation care and the discharge from observation. Note that you would not code the office visit because the office visit grew into a larger, more global service, i.e., the observation.

Hospital Inpatient Services

The Hospital Inpatient Services subsection is divided into codes for Initial Hospital Care and those for Subsequent Hospital Care.

Initial Hospital Care codes are for use by the admitting physician only. This may seem a bit awkward for you if your physician is not the admitting physician but is treating the patient.

Let's say the admitting physician is a cardiologist who is treating the patient for cardiovascular disease. Let's also say your doctor is an ophthalmologist who is seeing the patient for diabetic retinopathy. Because the ophthalmologist is not the physician who admitted the patient to the hospital, **CPT** explains that it would not be appropriate for him to use Initial Hospital Care codes. He would have to use Consultation codes or those for Subsequent Hospital Care.

Even though your physician is making the "initial" visit for **his** services, the use of Initial Hospital Care codes by a non-admitting physician is not correct according to **CPT**.

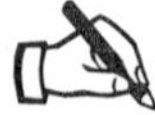

Remember: *If your physician admits the patient to the hospital on the same day as a hospital observation service is performed, use only the hospital admission code to report both services.*

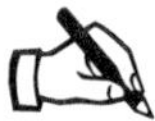

Remember: *If your physician saw the patient in an office/outpatient setting and decided at that visit to admit the patient to the hospital that day, be sure to use an Initial Hospital Care code for the admission,* ***not*** *an Office/Outpatient Visit code. All Evaluation and Management services provided to the patient on the same day are considered initial hospital care services.*

Subsequent Hospital Care codes include the following services:

- Review of the medical record;
- Review of diagnostic test results; and
- Observation and review of changes in the patient's status.

The same rules that are used in coding an Evaluation and Management service for an office visit also apply to all other Evaluation and Management services (e.g., how to pick a particular level of service by individually considering the kind of history, exam and medical decision making made). However, make sure that you read all the information given under the subheadings in your **CPT** book as it may give some additional helpful information about the codes that you did not know before.

At the end of the Hospital Inpatient Services subsection, under Hospital Discharge Services, are codes 99238 and 99239. These are the numbers used for coding the hospital discharge if it occurs on a different date than the hospital admission.

As you examine the codes below, note that they give a time frame for which the physician must perform the service.

99238	*Hospital discharge day management; 30 minutes or less*
99239	*Hospital discharge day management; more than 30 minutes*

The times illustrated in the code include the total amount of time that the physician needs (spends) to discharge the patient. This time can include the final exam of the patient, any counseling to the patient and/or family, preparation of prescriptions, referral forms, discharge records, and any other similar service that is directly related to discharging the patient. The total time spent to provide these services does not have to be continuous.

CONSULTATIONS

The subsection on consultations is probably the most difficult to understand in Evaluation and Management. Experience has shown that most coders are used to thinking of a consultation as a visit or service one physician provides to a patient on behalf of another physician — that is, the second physician looks at or treats the patient and then sends the patient back to the first physician. This is only partly true.

CPT is very clear about what is, in fact, a consultation. According to **CPT**, a consultation is a service provided by a physician at the request of another physician (or other appropriate source) whose opinion or advice regarding the treatment of the patient is sought for the further evaluation and/or management of the patient.

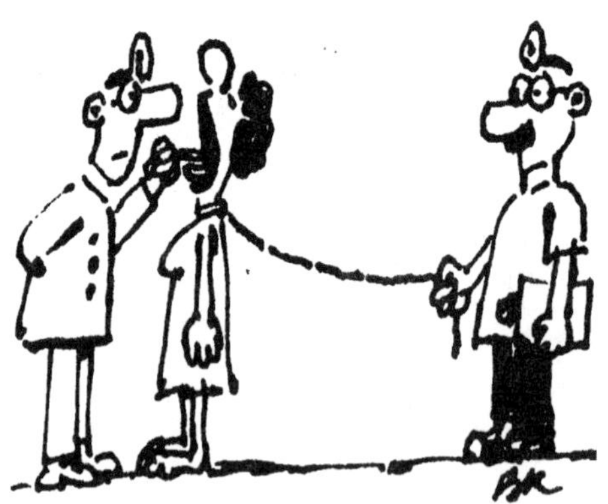

Consultation: Notice that the primary physician still has control (in this case with a leash) over the patient.

Notice that the first physician is not asking the second one to *treat* the patient (at least not at first). In other words, the *purpose* of the visit is not for treatment but rather to get the opinion or advice of the second doctor on how the first one *should treat* the patient.

These are instances, however, in which the patient will present to the "consultant" and it will be decided at that time (the time of the consultation) that "treatment" will begin. If we look at the purpose of the visit, we can see that the patient was sent to the consultant to get an opinion even though, in the end, the patient ended up starting treatment. In this case, the **CPT** book says you can still code for the consultation.

Consider this example. Let's say that a pediatrician notices that a six-year old patient seems to be slightly bowlegged. The pediatrician tells that patient's mother that she should take the child over to the orthopedist to see what, if anything, should be done. The mother makes an appointment with the orthopedist (the consultant in this case), who takes x-rays and completes an examination and history of the patient. Upon the completion of the visit, the orthopedist suggests that it may be helpful to use a special sole on the patient's shoes, and he actually writes down both the type of sole to be ordered and gives the mother the name of a qualified orthopedic shoe place where the special soles and/or shoes can be purchased. The orthopedist is confident that with this type of shoe the pediatrician can follow the patient and that there will be no additional need for the patient to return barring any other problems. The orthopedist writes a letter to the "referring" physician thanking her for the referral and points out his recommendations as well as the prescription and follow-through plans for the patient. Note in this case the orthopedist did not plan to treat the patient (the purpose of the visit was to tell the mother and her pediatrician if, in fact, there was a problem, i.e., to render an opinion). Once the patient was diagnosed and a simple remedy was available, the orthopedist made the prescription for the soles/shoes and sent the patient back with no expectations of continuing treatment of the six-year old.

This orthopedist can clearly, according to **CPT**, code for the consultation as the book tells us that a physician consultant may initiate diagnostic or therapeutic (as was done in this example) services.

Notice in the example above that the consulting physician should document in the patient's chart and communicate to the attending physician (in writing) the following information:

- Who requested the consultation;
- What tests were ordered or performed;
- What the diagnosis is, (e.g., the consultant's opinion);
- What treatment is recommended or performed.

Once the consulting physician assumes responsibility for the patient's continuing care, any subsequent service rendered by that physician is not a consultation.

hint

In order to use a consultation code in an office/outpatient setting, your physician must have seen the patient ***only for the*** *"**purpose**" of rendering an opinion.*

In other words, the next visit would not be a consultation but would be an office/outpatient visit, hospital visit, etc. The key here is whether the attending physician retains control over management of the patient's care or the patient's care is assumed by the consulting physician.

REFERRALS AND CONCURRENT CARE

To elaborate on the discussion above, the purpose of a consultation is to render an opinion or advice. Once the consulting physician takes over the patient's care, the patient has been *referred* to the consulting physician and now becomes his or her patient for the total or specific treatment of the problem(s). At least, that is the way insurance carriers use the word "refer."

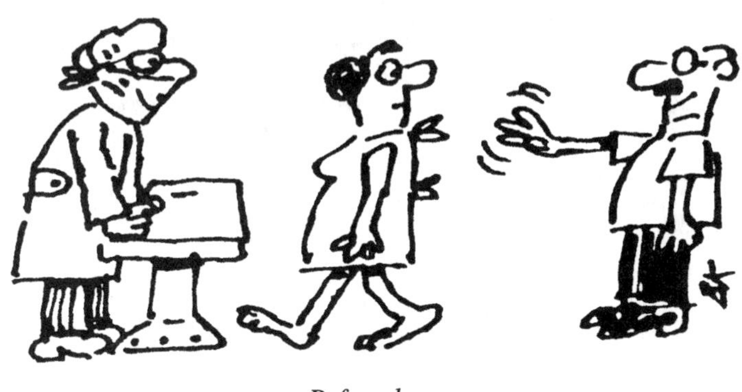

Referral

Physicians use the term "referral" the same way, but they also use it to describe a situation in which one physician sends a patient to another for the second physician's opinion. In other words, they use it to describe what insurance carriers and **CPT** call a consultation. It's important for you, the coder, to understand that for coding purposes, "referral" means the *transfer* of care and "consultation" means care provided to *render* *an opinion* (although, sometimes during a consultation, the physician does treat the patient).

At times, the consulting physician does not take over **complete** care of the patient from head to toe but assumes care regarding that portion for which he or she is qualified by specialty (e.g., the eyes or the bones). If the patient's original physician continues to treat the patient for another condition, the two physicians are now rendering concurrent care.

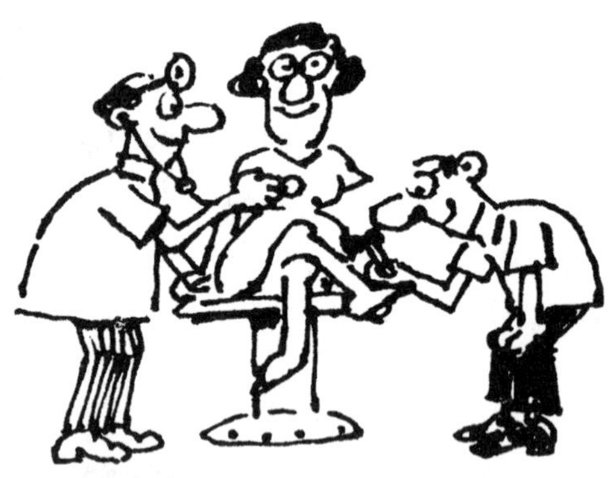

Concurrent care - two or more physicians "acting in conjunction"

Webster defines "concurrent" in the following way:

> ***"concurrent"*** *(kan-kur-rent) a. acting in conjunction; agreeing; taking place at the same time."*

Concurrent care is care (treatment) of the patient by two or more physicians (probably of different specialties) who are "acting in conjunction" with each other for the betterment of the patient's condition. In former versions of **CPT**, modifier -75 was used to indicate "concurrent care." This modifier no longer exists.

Notice that the "concurrent care" physician is not rendering complete care of the patient; he or she is treating only one or some of the patient's problems. However, this physician is still caring for (treating) the patient, rather than simply rendering an opinion (which would be the case under the definition of "consultation"). These visits would be considered "regular" visits (e.g., Office/Outpatient visits or Hospital Inpatient visits performed) on a concurrent care basis.

In the example we used before of the six-year old patient, had the orthopedist continued to treat the patient (e.g., had the patient returned for continued follow-up), the orthopedist would no longer be able to code using consultation codes but would have to use the Office/Outpatient visit codes found in the beginning of the Evaluation and Management Section.

You will see when you look at the Consultation codes that they are divided into four kinds of consultations:

- Office or Other Outpatient Consultations
- Initial Inpatient Consultations
- Follow-Up Inpatient Consultations
- Confirmatory Consultations

Let's look at each of these now.

Office or Other Outpatient Consultations: New or Established Patients

Office or Other Outpatient Consultations are visits during which the physician sets out to render his or her opinion in an office or outpatient setting.

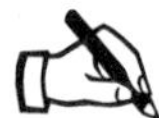

Remember: *The hospital, nursing facility or observation unit may qualify as an outpatient setting if the patient has not yet been admitted.*

This kind of consultation can occur in an emergency room (since the patient has not been admitted to the hospital), a physician's office, the observation area of a hospital, or any other place where a patient might be seen before admission to a hospital or nursing facility.

You will see that this series of codes, 99241 through 99245, is used for both new and established patients. In other words, if your physician's opinion or advice is requested on the same or a different problem, you can use these codes again and again.

It may be easier for you to understand the use and purpose of consultation codes if you know for sure when a consultation stops being a consultation (i.e., when you should switch from consultation codes to other codes). For example, let's say a patient went to a family practitioner (and had been seeing the family practitioner for years) and complained constantly of lower back pain. The family practice doctor may request that a neurosurgeon review the records of the patient, see the patient and render an opinion about the patient's back. If the neurosurgeon decided at the time of the consultation that the patient could benefit from physical therapy and traction and if the neurosurgeon actually prescribed this to the patient, **CPT** says that the neurosurgeon could still code a consultation.

Here is another example: Let's say a patient is sent to your office by the internal medicine doctor down the hall. Your physician's opinion has been requested because the patient failed to respond to the treatment the internal medicine doctor prescribed. After examining the patient, your physician concludes that his symptoms could mean one of two disorders. She puts him on a regimen and requests that he return in one week to see whether a firm diagnosis can be established. When the patient returns a week later he has not responded to the regimen, so your physician decides to run more tests. As you can see, both services are consultations. Why? Because your physician's opinion has been requested, and she has not yet reached a definitive diagnosis.

If your physician had arrived at a diagnosis during the first encounter and *had* begun treatment, the *second* (or next visit) would not have been considered a consultation but rather a regular office/outpatient visit. The **CPT** book explains that if the physician who performed the consulting sees the patient following the initial visit for "follow-ups" (which for us would be "treatment"), then the use of the Office/

Outpatient visits should be employed (if the service occurred in an office setting) or the subsequent hospital care codes should be used (if the service occurred in a hospital setting).

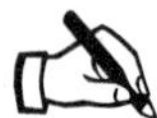

Remember: *As with everything else in the Evaluation and Management Section ...* ***You must document the need for your services!***

INITIAL INPATIENT CONSULTATIONS: NEW OR ESTABLISHED PATIENTS

CPT lists special codes for consultations rendered in an inpatient setting. There are two kinds of inpatient consultations:

- Initial Inpatient Consultations
- Follow-up Inpatient Consultations

Initial Inpatient Consultation codes (99251 through 99255) are used to report Initial Consultations on patients who have been admitted to a hospital or a nursing facility.

The inpatient consultation concept is a little different than the office/outpatient concept in that the **CPT** book gives the coder permission to use the Initial Inpatient Consultation code(s) when the "consulting" doctor sees the patient for a partial or complete transfer of care (e.g., they still allow you to code for a consultation even though you may be receiving the patient for treatment).

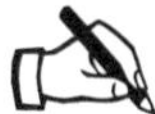

Remember: an initial inpatient consultation may take place in a hospital or a nursing facility and may be used ***for the first visit*** *when the patient comes to the doctor for the transfer of part or all of the care.*

FOLLOW-UP INPATIENT CONSULTATIONS: ESTABLISHED PATIENTS

Like Initial Inpatient Consultations, Follow-up Inpatient Consultations occur in hospitals and nursing facilities.

As its name implies, the Follow-up Consultation takes place when the consulting physician:

- Needs to complete an initial consultation; or
- Is called back to render an opinion on another problem for the same patient.

Let's take an example. Say your physician is asked to see a hospitalized patient for his opinion of an infection on the patient's elbow. He sees the patient and prescribes a course of therapy. He documents the visit in the patient's chart, communicates his findings to the attending physician, and leaves. Two weeks later, he is called back to see the same patient. This time, however, he is checking the patient and rendering his opinion to the primary physician for a different problem.

For the second consultation you would *not* use "Initial" Inpatient Consultation codes, even though your physician saw the patient for a different problem. You would use Follow-up Inpatient Consultation codes, because the patient had not been discharged from the hospital between the first and second times your physician saw him. Both consultation visits were made during the same hospital admission.

You could also use the Follow-up Inpatient Consultations codes if a physician sees the patient a second (third, fourth) time for the same problem. The determining factor on whether or not to use the subsequent consultations versus the initial is not to look at "why" the physician saw the patient so much as to look at "if" the second or third visits were during the same admission cycle as the Initial Inpatient Consultation visit.

Like Subsequent Hospital Care codes, Follow-up Inpatient Consultation codes include:

- Monitoring the patient's progress;
- Recommending to the attending physician a course of management (treatment) for the patient; and
- Advising the attending physician of any new plans

As with all kinds of consultations, once the physician reaches his or her diagnosis and treatment begins, **all subsequent services** for that problem are considered follow-up hospital visits or established patient nursing facility visits, rather than follow-up inpatient consultations.

Confirmatory Consultations: New or Established Patients

Confirmatory Consultation codes are used for second opinions. Anyone can request a second opinion (e.g., the patient or the insurance carrier), and many insurance companies now require them for surgeries. The carrier usually pays for confirmatory consultations. If the result of the confirmatory consultation is that surgery is NOT needed, the company has saved themselves and the patient the cost of the surgery. Codes 99271 through 99275 are used for confirmatory consultations.

If a carrier has required one of your patients to get a second opinion before a particular treatment can be rendered, you may consider using modifier -32 after the Confirmatory Consultation code you select to indicate that the second opinion was required or mandated (see Chapter Eleven: Modifiers). Confirmatory Consultations can occur anywhere; they are not limited to a particular treatment setting, as are Hospital Inpatient and Office/Outpatient Consultations. They also do not have typical time frames associated with the codes.

Let's take an example. A patient comes into your office that has been sent by a pediatrician. Both the mother and father are slightly distraught because it appears as if the last person they went to see about their son said that he HAD to have surgery and they just can't see that happening at this time. Both parents state that the child, a five year-old patient, has had flat feet for as long as they can remember but that he can run normally and plays like a regular kid. The orthopedist orders x-rays of both feet and examines the patient's

Example 6.5

DOC FORM

	OFFICE/OUTPATIENT		CONSULTATION	
	New(3)	Established(2)	Office/O.P.(3)	Confirm(3)
Minimal service		99211		
HISTORY				
Problem-Focused	99201	99212	99241	99271
Exp/Prob-Focused	99202	99213	99242	99272
Detailed	99203	99214	99243	99273
Comprehensive	99204/5	99215	99244/5	99274/5
EXAMINATION				
Problem-Focused	99201	99212	99241	99271
Exp/Prob-Focused	99202	99213	99242	99272
Detailed	99203	99214	99243	99273
Comprehensive	99204/5	99215	99244/5	99274/5
MEDICAL DECISION-MAKING				
Straight-Forward	99201/2	99212	99241/2	99271/2
Low Complexity	99203	99213	99243	99273
Mod Complexity	99204	99214	99244	99274
High Complexity	99205	99215	99245	99275
TIME: Total ______		Counsel/Coord. of Care:		______
10 minutes	99201	99212		
15		99213	99241	
20	99202			
25		99214		
30	99203		99242	
40		99215	99243	
45	99204			
60	99205		99244	
80			99245	

Patient Name: ______________________________

Date: __________ Physician's Signature: ______________________

MedBooks 101 West Buckingham, Richardson, Texas 75081

1-800-443-7397

www.medbooks.com

feet and legs completing a problem-focused history and an expanded problem-focused exam with medical decision-making of Low Complexity. Everyone is on board about the fact that this physician is being asked his opinion to either confirm or deny that this little boy needs surgery. Upon completion of the visit, the physician states that the boys condition can, most likely, be improved significantly by wearing good shoes and she prescribes a special type of shoe for the boy to wear. The parents leave (greatly relieved I might add) thanking the doctor for her services.

If you were to code this case using the DOC form, you would first look under the heading for Consultations. Under this heading, you would see several different kinds of consultations available for you to choose. In this case, since the consultation was a confirmatory one, you would select the column that is titled "confirm". Under that column, you would begin circling the code for Problem-Focused History and Expanded Problem-Focused Exam as well as the code that describes medical decision-making of Low Complexity.

As you can see by looking at the DOC form (see Example 6.5), you would have circled three different codes as follows:

A. the history, 99271

B. the exam, 99272 and

C. the medical decision making, 99273

The code you would select for the Mvaluation and Management service would be the code 99271 because, as is indicated by the number "3" following the word "confirm", you have to meet or exceed the highest common denominator three out of the three times. In this case, the code that you at least met or exceeded in all three instances would be the code 99271. It is important to note here that the code selection could have changed had the physician done more than a Problem-Focused History.

Emergency Department Services: New or Established Patients

Emergency Department Service codes range from 99281 through 99285. As with Confirmatory Consultation codes, no average time frames are provided with Emergency Department Service codes.

Here is an example:

99281 *Emergency department visit for the evaluation and management of a patient, which requires these three key components:*

- *a problem-focused history;*
- *a problem-focused examination; and*
- *straightforward medical decision-making.*

Counseling and/or coordination of care with other providers or agencies are provided consistent with the nature of the problem(s) and the patient's and/or family's needs.

Usually the presenting problem(s) are self-limited or minor.

The use of Emergency Department Service codes is limited to the reporting of services that occur in an emergency facility. An emergency facility is defined as:

- An organized hospital-based facility;
- Whose main function is to provide services to persons who have unscheduled events or are in need of immediate medical attention; and
- That is available 24 hours a day.

You must remember that in many emergency room situations, patients may present themselves in a crisis situation that may require surgery or some other form of treatment (e.g., car accident victim requiring repair of fractures). The Emergency Department Service codes only include the evaluation and management of the problem and *not* any procedures (e.g., x-ray, EEGs, surgeries etc.). These services (if provided) would be coded in addition to the Emergency Department Services. The use of the modifier -57 Decision for Surgery, or -25 Significant Separately Identifiable Evaluation and Management Service by the Same Physician on the Day of a Procedure, may be appropriately added to the Emergency Department Service codes. It is not the purpose of this chapter, however, to discuss modifiers, so we won't talk any more about them until we get to Chapter Eleven: Modifiers.

Selection of codes from the Emergency Department Services subsection requires the same process as selection of codes from other subsections we have discussed. It is based on the key components: history, examination, and medical decision-making.

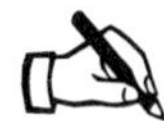

Emergency Department Services codes require that all three key components listed under the code be met.

CRITICAL CARE SERVICES

You will note when you look at the **CPT** book in the Critical Care section that quite a bit about it has changed over the past few years. The first thing that you may notice is that the entire Critical Care section has been subdivided into various other sections that include the following:

a. Transport of the pediatric critically ill or injured patient under 24 months of age;

b. Critical care services of non pediatric patients over the age of 24 months;

c. Critical care for pediatric patients over 31 days of age;

d. Critical care for pediatric patients under the age of 31 days (e.g., 30 days or less)

Beginning with the Pediatric Critical Care Patient Transport Section the **CPT** book addresses how to move a pediatric patient (under the age of 24 months) from one location to another. You will note that **CPT** has a special subsection dedicated especially to these cases (see 99289 – 99290). We will discuss more specifics on this in a few minutes. From here, the **CPT** book literally skips to what I call the regular critical care services (99291 - 99292) that basically outline how you would code for the care of a critically ill or critically injured non-pediatric patient. (You would think that since they start off with the "transport" of the critically ill or injured pediatric patient that they would continue with the "care" of the critically ill or injured patient but this is not the case.) After they have the discussed the "care" of a critically ill or injured non-pediatric patient, the books skips back again to talk about the "care" of the critically ill or injured "pediatric" patient (over the age of 31 days but up to 24 months of age, see 99293 - 99294) and then concludes with a subsection on critical care for neonates less than 31 days of age (i.e., 30 days or less), see 99295 - 99296.

In other words, it follows the following format:

a. Pediatric critical care patient transport

b. Critical care services

c. Neonatal and pediatric critical care services

   1. Pediatric critical care

   2. Neonatal critical care

   3. Intensive(non-critical) low birth weight services

Now let us take a brief look at each of these subsections.

Pediatric Critical Care Patient Transport

The subsection on patient transport was new to the **CPT** book for 2002. Basically, this subsection gives us a way to code for times when a physician must escort a critically ill or injured *pediatric* patient to another treatment facility. As you will see in other subsections of Evaluation and Management, the codes found here (99289 and 99290) allow the physician to be compensated for the "time" that was spent face-to-face with the pediatric patient (as opposed to the service of a history, exam and medical decision-making).

The 99289 code suggests that the physician spent somewhere between 30 minutes to 74 minutes taking the pediatric patient to the next facility. The 99290 code is used for each additional 30-minute time frame after the initial 74 minutes. Both codes suggest that the pediatric patient is 24-months of age or less.

For example, let's say the doctor started his/her constant face-to-face attendance with the patient from the maternity ward in a small town to the neonatology unit in the big city. Let's also say the time it took to actually assume responsibility for the patient at the maternity ward, transport the patient and surrender the baby to the next unit where responsibility for the patient is accepted was two hours (it was a long flight). In coding for this physician, you would code both the 99289 for the first 74 minutes and then the 99290 twice for the next 46 minutes. (The first 99290 would account for the first 30 minutes following the initial 74 minutes we got from the code 99289, and the second 99290 would account for the additional 16 minutes needed to get to the facility and get the baby checked in.) Notice that the physician cannot code for the return visit back to the maternity ward even though it will take him/her an additional two hours to get home. The codes 99289 and 99290 are not set up that way.

Also notice that during that flight, the physician may have to take the patient's pulse, monitor the patient's blood pressure and even, perhaps, give the patient some oxygen (e.g., mechanical ventilation). These services are considered "routine" and are not coded separately and are in addition to the codes for the transport. If, however, the physician had to do something that is not considered "routine" (e.g., setting up an IV drip (e.g., 90780, 90781) or performing CPR), the physician may code and bill for these services in addition to the codes for the transport.

NEONATAL AND PEDIATRIC CRITICAL CARE SERVICES

The purpose behind these codes is to provide the physician with a way of reporting his or her care of the critically ill infant or newborn or managing the intensive care of the very low birth weight infant of 30 days of age or less or in the intensive care unit.

General care includes:

- Management of the baby;
- Monitoring and treatment of the patient's nutrition (enteral and parental) metabolic and hematologic maintenance;
- Respiratory, pharmacologic control of the circulatory system;
- Parental/family counseling;
- Case management;
- Direct supervision of all nurses and other staff who are with the patient;
- Endotracheal intubation;
- Lumbar puncture;
- Suprapubic bladder aspiration.
- Oral or nasogastic tube placement;
- Bladder catheterization;
- Initiation and management of mechanical ventilation or continuous positive airway pressure (CPAP);
- Surfactant administration;
- Intravascular fluid administration;

- Umbilical venous and umbilical arterial, central, peripheral vessel or other arterial catheterization;
- Transfusion of blood components;
- Vascular punctures;
- Invasive or non-invasive electronic monitoring of vital signs;
- Bedside pulmonary function testing;
- Monitoring or interpretation of blood gases or oxygen saturation.

Other services that are listed under the specific Neonatal Intensive Care code and description are also included with the service for that particular code. For example consider the following **CPT** code.

99295 *Initial neonatal intensive care, per day, for the evaluation and management of a critically ill neonate or infant*

This code is reserved for the date of admission for neonates who are critically ill. Critically ill neonates require cardiac and/ or respiratory support (including ventilator or nasal CPAP when indicated), continuous or frequent vital sign monitoring, laboratory and blood gas interpretations, follow-up physician reevaluations, and constant observation by the health care team under direct physician supervision. Immediate preoperative evaluation and stabilization of neonates with life threatening surgical or cardiac conditions are included under this code. Neonates with life threatening surgical or cardiac conditions are included under this code. Care for neonates who require an intensive care setting but who are not critically ill is reported using the initial hospital care codes (99221-99223)

As you can see from the *description* of the code, services such as vital sign monitoring are included with the code *as well as* the services listed in the listed provided above. Services not listed in either the description of the code or above the description of the codes (in the notes) are not included with the codes themselves. An example would be closure of the septal defect of the heart or x-ray of the chest. You can also see by looking at the description of the code that it can be used once per day.

Other codes (e.g., physician standby, 99360, attendance at delivery 99436 and newborn resuscitation 99440) can be used in addition to the codes for neonatal critical care when the physician is present for the delivery and newborn resuscitation is required.

Note that although these codes are found in the Evaluation and Management Section, they do not mimic the usual codes found under the Evaluation and Management Section where different kinds of histories, examinations, and medical decision-making are described.

hint

Use of a particular code in the neonatal critical care unit is limited to one per day.

Pediatric Critical Care in this subsection of Evaluation and Management implies that the pediatric patient has either an acute injury or illness (e.g., central nervous system failure, circulatory failure, shock, and/or renal, hepatic, metabolic and/or respiratory failure) that can be fatal (or potentially fatal) if left untreated. It implies a crisis mode for both the patient and the physician and as such demands a high level of cognitive skills to assess, diagnosis, support, treat and/or prevent further deterioration of the patient's condition. If the condition of the patient is not as described above, you should not use these Pediatric Critical Care codes.

CRITICAL CARE SERVICES: TRANSPORT AND CARE OF NON PEDIATRIC PATIENTS

Critical Care, a subsection that many coders are unaware of, includes codes that describe the care of any person over the age of 24 months who is in a life-or-death situation, or one in which the illness or injury could really hurt one or more of the patient's vital organs (e.g., central nervous system failure, circulatory failure, shock, renal, hepatic, metabolic, and/or respiratory failure), thereby compromising their survival. This could be someone who suffers a heart attack or who has been in an auto accident. In general, critical care is needed in a situation when an individual's life or body part is threatened.

The Critical Care codes apply to patients who are at least 24 months old. If the patient is younger than 24 months of age, and critical care is performed, you should use the codes for neonatal or pediatric intensive care.

Notice that critical care is not always given in a critical care setting such as the Intensive Care Unit, or Critical Care Unit. These codes (99291 and 99292) can be used any time a physician performs certain procedures on an unstable individual to save the person's life, no matter what the location or setting. These codes would not apply when the physician transports the critically ill or injured patient. For those instances, use the patient transport codes (99289 and 99290).

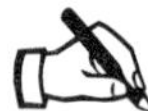

Remember: *Unlike the transport codes for patients under age 24 months who are critically ill or injured (see 99290), there are no "special codes" for "transport" of critically ill or injured patients over the age of 24 months. Use the codes 99291 – 99292 when you provide critical care and/or transport of these non-pediatric patients.*

Critical care codes are based solely on time rather than on the kind of history, examination and medical decision making involved. When providing critical care, the physician gives constant attention to the patient in the sense that the physician is providing services that are directly related to that patient's care (e.g., reviewing lab tests, monitoring cardiac output measurements, discussing the patient's condition to staff, family members or guardians, etc.). These codes take the following services into account:

- Interpretation of cardiac output measurements
- Pulse oximetry
- Chest x-rays
- Blood, gases, and information stored in computers
- Temporary transcutaneous pacing
- Gastric intubation
- Ventilator management
- Vascular access procedures

Services performed which are not listed above should be reported separately.

For example, if the physician performs CPR on a patient with a heart attack, as well as the services listed above, the CPR is coded separately in addition to the code for the critical care. It is NOT included in the critical-care time (notice that it's not part of the list above). If the physician takes a chest x-ray during critical-care time or takes cardiac output measurements, these *would* be included in the critical-care time and would not be coded separately. If the physician has to suture the patient, reduce a fracture, or anything else that is not directly related to stabilization, these services must be coded separately.

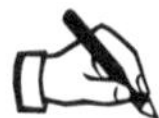

Critical care codes are those used in life-threatening situations in which the physician is in constant attendance of the unstable, critically ill/injured patient.

CPT lists two critical care codes: 99291 for the first 30 - 74 minutes of critical care and 99292 for each subsequent 30 minutes of critical care.

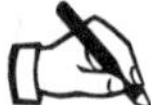

Remember *that all critical care your physician renders on a particular day for a given patient should be reported by adding up all of the time for that day and reporting it in total, as described above. Code 99291 should only be used once per day.*

If your physician performed critical care for two hours, you would code the procedure by placing 99291 in the **CPT/HCPCS** column on the HCFA claim form and 1 in the Units column. To show the second hour, you would place 99292 in the **CPT/HCPCS** column and 2 in the Units column (1/2 hour plus 1/2 hour = 1 hour). If the duration of the critical care service was an hour and a half, the service would be coded using 99291 for the first hour and 99292 for the next half hour, with 1 in each of the Units columns.

Once critical care has taken place for a given day, subsequent critical care on a different day can be reported with the use of the same codes again.

On a final note, conversations that have a direct relationship to the management of the patient (i.e., the patient is "out cold" and/or is unable to participate or incompetent), the time the physician spends on the floor or in the critical care unit with decision

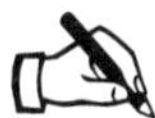

Also remember this: *If your physician provides services to a patient in the critical care area, but the patient is not "critically ill" or the services are not critical care services meant to stabilize him or her, the appropriate hospital visit codes or other procedure codes (rather than critical care codes) should be used.*

makers (e.g., family) can be added up as part of the overall critical care time.

INTENSIVE (NON-CRITICAL) LOW BIRTH WEIGHT SERVICES

Let's suppose that you are a pediatrician (or neonatologist) who has had a patient in the critical care unit for a variety of problems which have now been stabilized. Let's further suppose that this patient is not yet ready to go home because it is still extremely small but that it no longer needs the services of the critical care unit. **CPT** has developed a subsection within the **CPT** book Evaluation and Management Section that you can use to describe services that would apply to these patients (see codes 99298 and 99299). Let's review these codes.

99298 *Subsequent intensive care, per day, for the evaluation and management of the recovering very low birth weight infant (present body weight less than 1500 grams)*

Infants with present body weight less than 1500 grams who are no longer critically ill continue to require intensive cardiac and respiratory monitoring, continuous and/or frequent vital sign monitoring, heat maintenance, enteral and/or parenteral nutritional adjustments, laboratory and oxygen monitoring and constant observation by the health care team under direct physician supervision.

99299 *Subsequent intensive care, per day, for the evaluation and management of the recovering low birth weight infant (present body weight 1500-2500 grams)*

Infants with present body weight of 1500-2500 grams who are no longer critically ill continue to require intensive cardiac and respiratory monitoring, continuous and/or frequent vital sign monitoring, heat maintenance, enteral and/or parenteral nutritional adjustments, laboratory and oxygen monitoring and constant observation by the health care team under direct physician supervision.

As you can see, these codes are different because they describe babies of different weight ranges. If the baby receives these intensive (but not "critical care type") services and the baby weighs less than 1500 grams, you would use the code 99298. If the baby weighs more than 1500 grams (from 1500 to 2500 grams) you would use the 99299 code.

Nursing Facility Services

The next subsection of Evaluation and Management covers nursing facility services. This subsection uses the same key components as other subsections: history, examination, and medical decision-making.

As its name implies, a nursing facility is one that employs professional (e.g., degreed) staff 24 hours a day. In these types of facilities, the physician has a role in ensuring that a medical plan for each patient is followed or revised to maintain or improve that patient's status.

There are two basic kinds of nursing facility services:

- Comprehensive Nursing Facility Assessment
- Subsequent Nursing Facility Care

A Comprehensive Nursing Facility Assessment may be provided when the patient is evaluated for admission to a nursing facility. They may also be provided to a patient who is already in a nursing facility.

A Comprehensive Nursing Facility Assessment can be made almost anywhere. For example, these assessments may take place in a doctor's office, a hospital, or an emergency room. Because these appraisals are performed in one of several locations, their coding can be confusing. For example, should you code for an office visit, or a nursing assessment, or both? If your physician is providing this Evaluation and Management service in a hospital as a condition for the patient's admission to a 24-hour, professionally staffed facility, you must only use the Evaluation and Management code for Comprehensive Nursing Facility Assessment. The only service that may be coded separately is the hospital discharge.

Subsequent Nursing Facility Care codes (99311 through 99313) describe E/M services provided to patients in a nursing facility. These codes are used for visits to patients who do not require comprehensive assessments or for those who have not experienced a major change in status. Just as you saw with the hospital inpatient visits and observation or inpatient care services, there are codes for the discharge from a nursing facility. See codes 99315 and 99316.

Domiciliary, Rest Home (e.g., Boarding Home) or Custodial Services

It is important to understand the differences between a nursing facility and a domiciliary, rest home, boarding home or custodial care service.

The basic purpose of a domiciliary, rest home, or boarding home is to provide a place for the patient to live, unlike the nursing facility where medical care is provided (e.g., dispensing of prescriptions). The presence of professional staff is not required, and patients may or may not be receiving therapy. You may have seen these homes popping up in your area since they are becoming increasingly popular residential choices for patients who are ambulatory and don't require a skilled level of care.

HOME SERVICES

The Home Service codes are similar to the other Evaluation and Management codes we have discussed. The important thing to remember here is that these codes apply only to services provided in the patient's private residence.

You may find the term "private residence" a bit vague, since some patients live in apartment-type settings with many other patients. If the patient receives the types of services that you receive at your private residence (e.g., mail direct from a postal carrier, especially bills for which the patient is responsible) and he or she prepares meals, the setting in all likelihood would qualify as the patient's private residence. If the patient does not receive these services, the residence is more apt to be a boarding facility or domiciliary.

You code home services by identifying the history, examination, and medical decision-making, as you do for other Evaluation and Management services. Keep in mind that a new patient visit will require at least three key components and an established patient visit will require at least two.

PROLONGED SERVICES

Codes found in the Prolonged Services subsection of Evaluation and Management describe procedures which go above and beyond the normal Evaluation and Management services for inpatient or outpatient settings.

As we discussed before, the regular office/outpatient services include histories, exams and decision-making processes regarding the treatment planning for the patient. Some counseling can also be considered part of the regular Evaluation and Management services. But what happens when the rest of the visit, the part after the history and medical decision exam, takes an extended period of time (more than 30 minutes)? In a case such as this, when an Evaluation and Management service is rendered to a patient but the treatment phase or the coordination of the treatment phase with relatives, friends or caregivers is longer than 30 minutes, the Prolonged Services codes can be used *in addition to* (note plus sign [✚] for "add-on code" status on the prolonged service codes in your **CPT** book) the codes for Evaluation and Management.

There are three kinds of Prolonged Services.

1. Face-to-face or direct patient contact;
2. Non-face-to-face (indirect) patient contact;
3. Physician standby services

Face-To-Face Prolonged Services

In the face-to-face prolonged service, the physician spends time with the patient one on one. There are two types of face-to-face prolonged services. These are the ones that occur in:

1. An Office/Outpatient setting
2. An inpatient setting

In both sites (office/outpatient or inpatient), the physician "treats" the patient. An example might be the evaluation, management and treatment of a patient who has gone into pre-term labor. The physician may administer Terbutaline/Brethine and then continue to monitor the patient for some time, making sure that both mom and baby are okay and that the patient's vital signs (blood pressure, pulse, etc.) remain stable. If the service of staying with the patient during this face-to-face monitoring of her treatment is more than 30 minutes, the physician may then code both the Evaluation and Management service for hospital observation or admission (whichever is appropriate) as well as the face-to-face prolonged service code for the treatment and monitoring of the patient. Note that the physician can leave and come back. What is coded, however, is the total duration of face-to-face time spent with the patient on a cumulative basis.

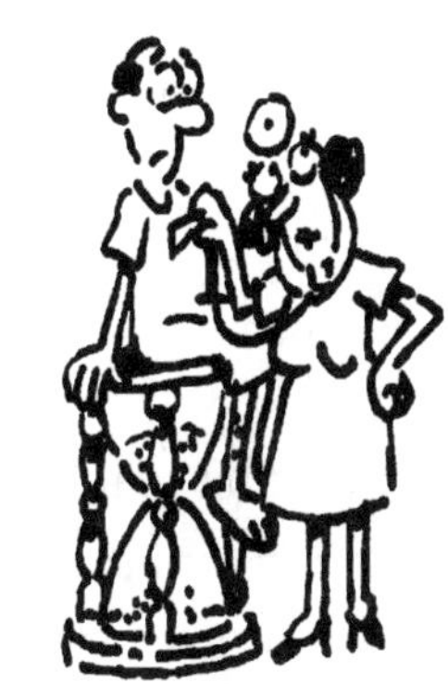

If the face-to-face treatment is more than 30 minutes, both the Evaluation and Management and Prolonged Service codes can be used.

Non-Face-To-Face Prolonged Service

To illustrate non-face-to-face prolonged services, let's consider the following example: Suppose that a patient is mentally impaired and has to be cared for by a relative or hired caregiver. The physician evaluates the patient in her office and discovers that in addition to her mental impairment, she appears to have a cold and flu and has recently become diabetic. Following the visit, the physician spends an extensive amount of time talking with the patient's care-giver, reviewing the medical records transferred from other physicians and completing an extensive treatment plan. The physician then coordinates the care plan with a local home health care agency and a dietician.

Notice that in this example the time spent non-face-to-face with the actual patient is more than simply counseling and/or coordination of care (as is already included in the normal Evaluation and Management services). In this case, the "time" was spent in the actual treatment of the patient (e.g., arranging care with the persons responsible for actually treating the patient).

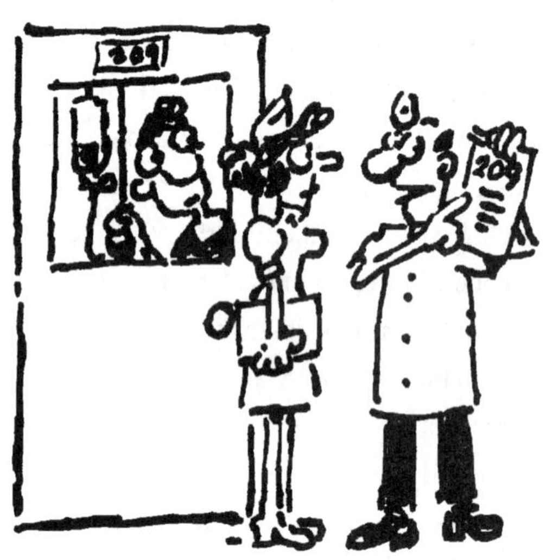

Patient is not present during the non-face-to-face monitoring of treatment.

Physician Standby Services

Physician standby is used when a physician spends time waiting for a service to occur (e.g., neonatologist waiting for a high-risk infant to be born or neurologist waiting for a patient to be stabilized before performing his or her nonsurgical neurologic procedures).

Consider how the code and description are written.

99360 *Physician standby service, requiring prolonged physician attendance, each 30 minutes (e.g., operative standby, standby for frozen section, for cesarean/high risk delivery, for monitoring EEG)*

Note that this code allows at least 30 minutes of monitoring. You could report this code twice if you had one hour of standby time, but you must make sure that the reason(s) for your wait are documented in the medical chart and that an additional full 30 minutes was spent waiting.

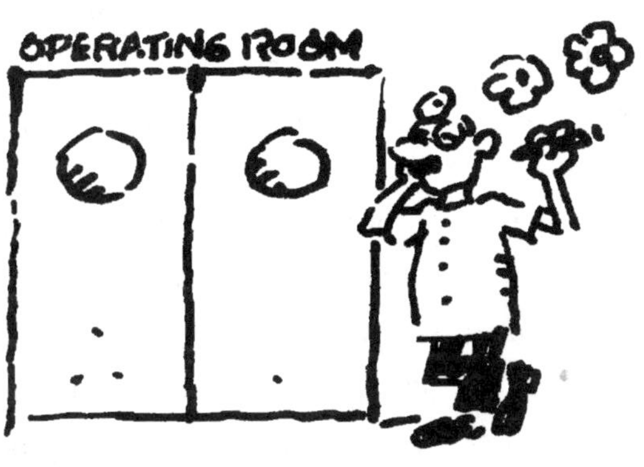

Physician Standby

If a physician stands by and waits for a surgery to be performed and then actually performs a surgery himself, the operative standby codes should not be used because the time spent waiting would be considered by **CPT** to be part of the Surgical Package.

If the physician is required to be on call at the hospital (as opposed to being "on-standby") because either the patient requested it or another physician requested it, the code 99360 should not be used. In cases where the physician is either on call or mandated by the hospital to be there (e. g., they may or may not be on "operative standby"), the codes 99026 and 99027 which describe hospital mandated or on call services should be employed. These codes can be found in the Medicine Section and will be discussed when we come to that chapter.

CASE MANAGEMENT SERVICES

Codes in this subsection (99361 through 99373) describe telephone calls and medical conferences. In prior versions of **CPT,** these codes were found in the Medicine Section.

This subsection provides physicians with a means of reporting the initiation, coordination, and supervision of health care services provided to patients. Case Management Services include talking with the lab about test results; discussing those results with the patient over the telephone; coordinating the patient's medical management with nurses, therapists, and other health care professionals; and discussing the treatment plan with the patient and/or family over the telephone.

Let's take a closer look at these codes.

99361 *Medical conference by a physician with interdisciplinary team of health professionals or representatives of community agencies to coordinate activities of patient care (patient not present); approximately 30 minutes*

99362 *approximately 60 minutes*

As you can see, these two codes are to be used when the physician confers with a team of health care professionals and the patient is absent.

The next three codes (99371, 99372, and 99373) are to be used for telephone calls. Code 99371 is for a brief phone call by the physician to the patient to report lab results, clarify or alter previous instructions, or adjust therapy.

Code 99372 is used for an intermediate phone call in which the physician provides advice to an established patient on a new problem, initiates therapy that can be started over the phone, discusses test results in detail, and other such services. For example, let's say that a patient's Pap smear comes out showing that the cells are inflamed. The physician may call the patient, explain the situation to her, and recommend that she get some Gynelotrimin and repeat the pap after she finishes the course of treatment.

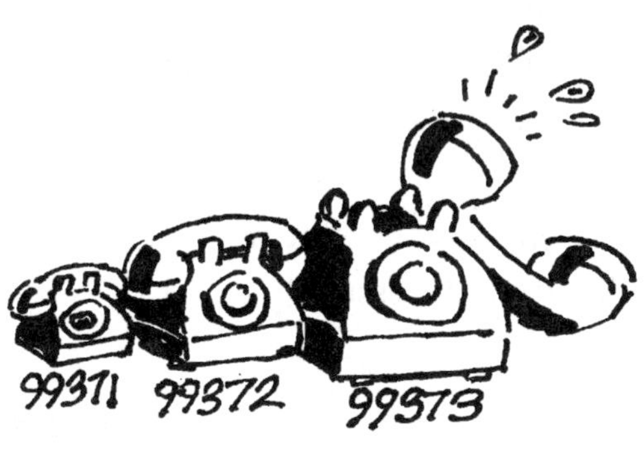

Code 99373 is used to describe a complex or lengthy phone call. You would use this code if you wanted to bill for a phone call to an anxious or distraught patient, a detailed or prolonged discussion with family members regarding a seriously ill patient, or any lengthy telephone communication necessary to coordinate the complex services of several health professionals charged with different aspects of the patient's total care plan. An example may be reporting the results of an HIV lab test which showed positive for HIV. Obviously the patient would be distraught and may require a significant amount of telephone assistance and counseling.

CARE PLAN OVERSIGHT SERVICES

This title is amusing at first glance as you might consider the oversight services to be some service that was overlooked. In this case however, oversight is the "overseeing of" the care of the patient and implies the physician setting up a 30-day care plan for the patient monitoring the patient's status through review of reports and lab tests, communication with others involved in the patient's care, and revising the treatment plan when necessary.

The patient may be under the direct care of a home health agency, hospice, or nursing facility when there is a need for supervision on a recurring basis by the physician. If the physician is not needed on a recurrent basis (e.g., the home health agency

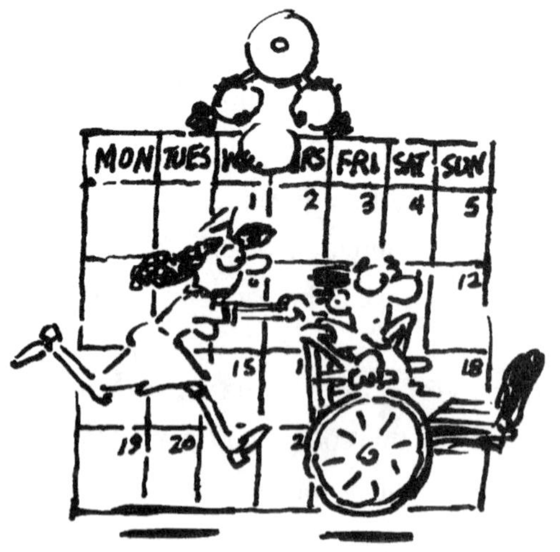

The physician oversees a 30-day care plan.

follows the doctor's orders over the period of time but does not need the physician to review lab results), to revise the action plan for the patient's case and communicate with other health professionals about the patient's status, then you would not use these codes but would include any labor intensive services with the home/office/outpatient visits, nursing or domiciliary visit codes.

As with some of the other codes found in the Evaluation and Management Section, the Care Plan Oversight services are coded based on the amount of time spent providing the service(s).

PREVENTIVE MEDICINE SERVICES

Webster defines the word "prevent" in the following way:

> ***'prevent"*** *"to keep from happening or existing; to deal with beforehand; getting ahead so as to stop or interrupt something in its course."*

The subsection on Preventive Medicine describes services rendered to a patient in order to keep problems from occurring (e.g., a routine gynecologic checkup or a visit to the pediatrician to weigh a normal, healthy infant). More often than not, the patient presents herself with no real medical complaint (e.g., no back pain, no sore throat, etc.).

The **CPT** book points out that if a problem is found during the Preventive Medicine visit that requires additional work necessitating the completion of an additional history, exam, and medical decision-making, the appropriate Office/Outpatient code may be used in addition to the code for Preventive Medicine. An example might be of someone who comes in for an annual physical (e.g., to make sure that all body systems are functioning properly and to hopefully "catch" any problem(s) in time that may have cropped up since the last visit). During the course of the exam you note that the patient has an arrythmia and appears to have congested lungs. Both of these conditions may require additional work on the part of the physician and would qualify her or him to also be able to bill out the Office/Outpatient visit (with a modifier -25 Significant, Separately Identifiable E/M Service By Same M.D. on Same Day appended to the end of it) *and* the Preventive Medicine code.

In general, Preventive Medicine Services are not generously reimbursed by many carriers. This is because most carriers do not pay for well care. Most seem to only reimburse physicians or patients for services rendered to alleviate a specific problem.

Preventive Medicine codes 99381 through 99397 include counseling or helping a patient to lower his or her risk of illness or injury (e.g., talking to the patient about current unhealthy habits such as smoking or overeating). They also include identification of risk factors (e.g., finding out that the patient has high blood pressure or that he or she smokes), the ordering of tests, and the history and examination.

Let's take a closer look at these codes.

99381 *Initial comprehensive preventative medicine evaluation and management of an individual including an age and gender appropriate history, examination, counseling/anticipatory guidance/risk factor reduction interventions, and the ordering of appropriate immunization(s), laboratory/diagnostic procedures, new patient; infant (age under 1 year)*

99382 *early childhood (age 1 through 4 years)*

As you can see, these Preventive Medicine services are separated by patient age going up to a **CPT** code for patients 65 years and older (see 99387 or 99397). There are separate codes for new patients and for established patients.

Counseling and/or Risk-Factor Reduction Intervention

These counseling and/or risk-factor reduction codes cannot be used for counseling if the patient already has symptoms or an established illness related to the risk factor (e.g., you can't use these codes if the patient already has emphysema and smokes and you are trying to get them to quit). These codes would be used if the counseling and/or risk-factor reduction session occurred as a separate encounter (not part of an

Office/Outpatient visit or Preventive Medicine Service). Say a 15-year-old patient came into the OB/GYN office to discuss the possibility of going on the pill. If this were a separate encounter not associated with a Preventive Medicine Service or Office/Outpatient Visit, it could be coded using these codes.

It makes sense that these codes would be used only for encounters that do not occur with or another type of space considered to be an observation area scheduled visit, i.e., they cannot be used together with a Preventive Medicine visit or an Office visit, etc. The reason for the "separate session" requirement is that counseling and or coordination of care are normal integral parts of regular E/M visits (e.g., counseling and/or coordination of care are already part of such visits as Office/Outpatient visits, Hospital Inpatient visits).

Notice that the Counseling and/or Risk-Factor Reduction Intervention codes list the amount of time spent with the patient as part of the description of the code. This time is important to denote in your chart will help you code the visit appropriately. It is also important to document the nature of the visit in your chart (e.g., what was discussed).

NEWBORN CARE

The Evaluation and Management sSection of **CPT** features a subsection of codes to be used for services provided to normal newborns. As you look through these codes, you will see that they describe the following services:

- Histories and examinations for newborns;
- Normal newborn care (not in hospital or birthing room);
- Hospital newborn care;
- Newborn resuscitation;
- Attendance at the delivery.

Use these codes rather than Office or Inpatient Visit codes for reporting all care for newborns whether the service occurs in the office/outpatient or inpatient basis.

SPECIAL EVALUATION AND MANAGEMENT SERVICES

This section (codes 99450 through 99456) was added to **CPT** in 1995. Basically, these codes are used to code for baseline evaluations to patients who need reports written on their behalf for the purpose of obtaining life insurance, disability insurance, or work-related medical disability forms. Notice as you read through these codes that no active treatment or management of the problem (if encountered) takes place. The sole purpose of the visits is to assess the patient's overall health and report findings accordingly.

CHECK YOUR CODE USAGE

Once you have mastered the Evaluation and Management Section, it would be a good idea to periodically check your code usage by plotting it on a graph. You can do this by drawing one line from north to south (top to bottom) which will mark the *number* of each kind of visit you have provided and then on a line on your page from left to right which will indicate the *kind* of visit (e.g., office/outpatient, new patient). After you have completed your graph, your results should show a wide bell-shaped curve similar to the one below.

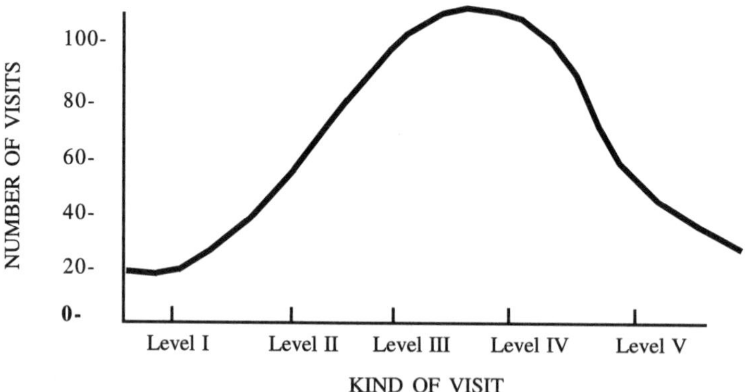

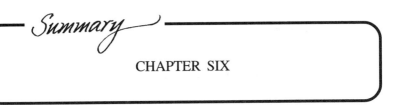

- ✓ The Evaluation and Management Section is the first section in **CPT, Current Procedural Terminology.**

- ✓ All codes in the Evaluation and Management Section begin with the number 9.

- ✓ Services found in the Evaluation and Management Section include histories, examinations, and decisions that must be made regarding the patient's diagnosis and treatment.

- ✓ A new patient is one who has not received any professional services from a physician or services from another doctor of the same specialty within the same group practice within the past three years. This definition also holds true for Medicare reporting.

- ✓ An established patient is one who has received professional services from a given physician or another physician of the same specialty and within the same group practice within the past three years.

- ✓ It is important to understand the four different kinds of histories, the four different kinds of examinations, and the variety of decisions that can be made before you try to use Evaluation and Management codes.

- ✓ Key components are conditions or elements that must be met to qualify for a particular service code.

- ✓ The three key components discussed in the Evaluation and Management Section are history, examination, and medical decision-making.

- ✓ To qualify for a particular Evaluation and Management code, most new patient visits require that all three key components be met or exceeded.

- ✓ To qualify for a particular Evaluation and Management code, most established patient visits require that only two of three key components be met or exceeded.

- ✓ Even though average time frames are listed in the descriptions of many Evaluation and Management codes, time usually is not a factor in selecting an appropriate code.

- ✓ Time is the deciding factor in choosing most Evaluation and Management codes when the counseling or coordination of care portion of the visit takes more than 50% of the total time spent with the patient.

✓ Hospital Observation Services are used to report histories, exams and medical decisions made on patients in an observation area of a hospital. This location could be a specialized observation unit, the emergency department or another type of space considered to be an observation area.

✓ Observation services are to be used on patients who receive services but who have not been admitted to the hospital.

✓ Initial Hospital Care codes can be used only by the admitting physician. All other physicians who provide initial hospital care must use either Consultation codes (if appropriate) or Subsequent Hospital Care codes.

✓ Consultations are defined as services in which the consulting physician is expected to render an opinion or give advice.

✓ If a physician treats a patient during a consultation at the request of the attending physician, the service qualifies as a consultation.

✓ If a physician treats a patient during a consultation, any *subsequent* service rendered by the consulting physician to that patient is considered an Evaluation and Management service **other than** a consultation (e.g., Office/Outpatient visit, Hospital visit) and should be coded accordingly.

✓ Emergency Department Service codes are to be used only when the service is rendered in a 24-hour hospital-based facility that specializes in providing treatment for unscheduled events.

✓ The Emergency Department Service codes do not include surgeries and many other procedures.

✓ Patient Transport codes 99289 and 99290 can only be used for face-to-face services provided by a physician who spends at least 30 minutes with a pediatric patient (24 months of age or less) who is critically ill or injured going from point A to point B. You can also code any nonroutine services done during that time.

✓ Critical Care codes describe services rendered at certain specified time frames to stabilize the unstable, critically ill or injured patient who is experiencing a life-threatening situation.

✓ There is a definitive difference in the coding of critical care services provided to neonates (children under 31 days of age) versus those who are from 31 days of age to 24 months of age. Likewise, there is also a difference in coding the critical care services from those two groups (i.e., neonates and pediatric cases under 24 months) and those critical care services rendered to patients older than 24 months of age.

✓ Critical Care codes include interpretation of cardiac output measurements, chest x-rays, pulse oximetry, blood gases, and information data stored in computers (e.g., ECG's, blood pressures), gastric intubation, temporary transcutaneous pacing, ventilator management and vascular access procedures. Services that are not part of this list should be coded separately.

✓ Nursing Facility Services can be further subdivided into two basic groups. Those services that include a comprehensive nursing facility assessment (where the patient is evaluated for admission to an nursing facility or assessed due to a change in their status) and those services that occur in a subsequent nursing facility where the patient is already a resident of such a facility and who has not experienced any change of status but whom the physician sees.

✓ A nursing facility is one that provides a 24-hour therapeutically planned and professionally staffed group living and learning environment. These facilities were formerly known as Skilled Nursing Facilities, Intermediate Care Facilities, or Long Term care Facilities.

✓ Home Services are those visits where the physician performs evaluation and management services to patients who are living in a private residence. These home services use different codes from those that occur in a domiciliary, rest home, boarding home or custodial care situation.

✓ Prolonged Services are those in which the "treatment" of the patient and/or the coordination of care involves at least a 30-minute period beyond the usual services.

✓ Prolonged Services have the add-on code notation and can be used in addition to the code for the Evaluation and Management service.

✓ Care Plan Oversight Services are those procedures in which a physician is integrally involved in overseeing and monitoring the care of patients for at least 30 days under the direct care of nursing homes or home health organizations. This may include physician development of a course of action, review of lab results, telephone calls, integration of new information into a plan of action, adjustment of therapy, etc..

✓ Preventive Medicine codes describe services provided to patients who desire to nip their problem(s) in the bud and in many cases have no specific complaints, problems, or established illnesses.

✓ The Counseling and/or Risk Factor Reduction codes cannot be used in conjunction with another E/M visit in which history, exam and medical decision-making are provided.

✓ Special Evaluation and Management services include examinations used to evaluate the health of the patient and get a baseline idea of the patient's physical status so that a disability or life insurance policy can be issued.

CHAPTER SEVEN

SURGERY

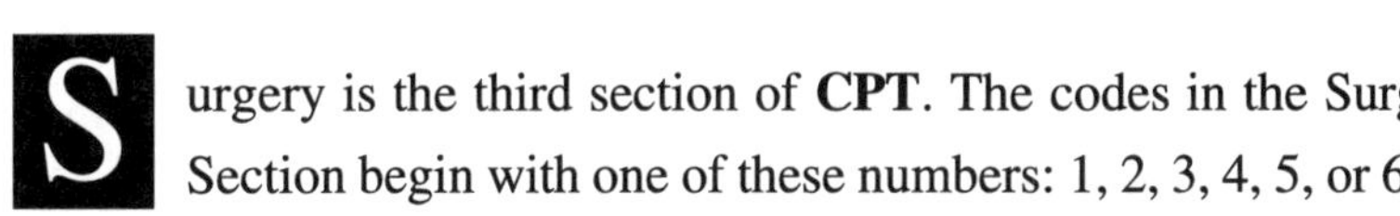

Surgery is the third section of **CPT**. The codes in the Surgery Section begin with one of these numbers: 1, 2, 3, 4, 5, or 6.

The majority of the Surgery Section is arranged from the outside to the inside of the body. If we were to cut through the body with a scalpel, the first organ we would encounter is the Integumentary System—the skin. This is the first subsection of the Surgery Section and these codes begin with the number 1.

The next structure or organ we would encounter is the Musculoskeletal System—the muscles and bones.

Accordingly, the Musculoskeletal System is the second subsection of the Surgery Section and these codes begin with the number 2.

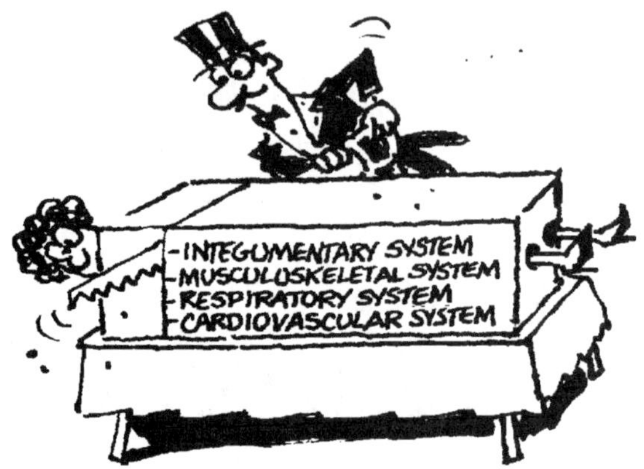

"Much of the Surgery Section is arranged from the outside to the inside of the body."

We would next find the Respiratory System — lungs. These codes begin with the number 3. Beneath the Respiratory System would be the Cardiovascular System — heart and blood vessels. These codes also begin with the number 3.

Not all of the Surgery Section is arranged from the outside of the body to the inside (we run out of structures after a while), but now you have the general idea.

Like the other sections, the Surgery Section begins with its own guidelines. These guidelines explain some of the nuances you will see in the Surgery Section.

Guidelines in the Surgery Section describe points that are very important to the comprehension of this section. It is essential that you read these guidelines point-by-point and understand each one completely before proceeding to the next.

Let's look at each guideline in detail. It would be helpful for you to grab a copy of **CPT,** turn to the Surgery Section guidelines and read along with the description of each guideline below.

PHYSICIANS' SERVICES

This guideline directs you to both the Evaluation and Management Section and the Medicine Section, where you will find codes for noninvasive services (special services and reports), and procedures (noninvasive cardiovascular, otorhinolaryngology, ophthalmology, and pathology procedures).

You will also find other noninvasive procedures — such as the histories and physicals performed in conjunction with the evaluative process used in arriving at a treatment plan — in the first section of **CPT**, Evaluation and Management. Noninvasive procedures found in the Evaluation and Management Section include such services as office/outpatient visits, hospital visits, and consultations.

SURGICAL PACKAGES

Listed surgical procedures in **CPT**, those that begin with the numbers 1, 2, 3, 4, 5, and 6 and are not followed by a star (**✱**), include:

SURGICAL PACKAGE

a. Local infiltration, metacarpal/metatarsal digital block or topical anesthesia when used.

b. One E/M service (directly related to the surgery) on the day of or the day before the surgery. This E/M service is **NOT** the one during which you decide to operate.

c. The operation per se.

d. Postoperative care including the dictation of the surgery (notes), the discussion with the patient and/or family of the surgical outcome and the follow-up treatment, the writing of the orders, evaluation of the patients and how they are recovering from anesthesia, and routine, normal follow-up care.

The 2002 version of **CPT** brought about a much clearer definition of what was included in the Surgical Package. This change, described above, was much more in line with what the carriers have stated the surgical package is and should prove to be a big help for anyone trying to follow the rules. Simply put, the Surgical Package means that each non-starred service between numbers one through six includes the local infiltration, digital block(s) or topical anesthesia provided before surgery as well as the Evaluation and Management visit that is required to make sure that the patient is still ready to undergo the surgery itself, and the normal, uncomplicated follow-up which includes the writing of your notes, the directions to the hospital staff if the patient is to remain in the hospital, the post-surgery conferences with the patient and/or family and the post-anesthesia recovery progress. It does not include the Evaluation and Management visit that the patient had when you first decided that surgery was necessary. In other words, the Surgical Package is similar to the "blue plate special" we talked about in Chapter Five. It includes everything for one price.

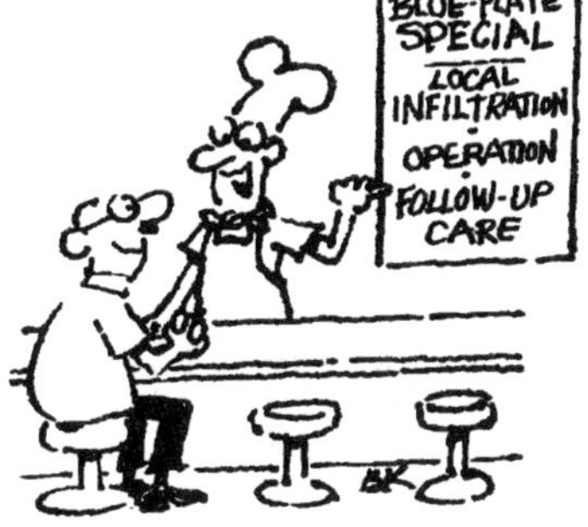

The Surgical Package is similar to the "blue plate special."

Here is an example of the Surgical Package. Let's say that someone came into your office with pain in her wrist. Upon examination and x-ray, together with the appropriate history, you find out that the patient has a soft tissue mass in her forearm. You conclude that the patient needs to have a biopsy of that soft tissue and inform the patient. You and the patient agree that the "surgery" (biopsy of the soft tissue of the forearm/wrist) should occur the following week. You code for the Evaluation and Management service rendered on that date.

When the day of the surgery arrives, you again reassess the patient's condition, making sure to note any changes that may have occurred. Essentially, you have performed another evaluation and management of the patient's condition. You decide that things are as they were a week ago and proceed with your plans to operate. You provide the appropriate anesthesia, perform the biopsy, bring the patient into recovery, dictate your notes and inform the family and the patient of the results. You advise the patient to return in one week to remove sutures and check the patient's progress. All of this, and more as the number of follow-up days that go with this procedure are 10 (see **Medicare RBRVS: A Physician's Guide**), is included in the price you charged for the surgery. You provided a package deal...a blue plate special.

The Surgical Package applies to all surgical codes except those in which a star (✱) follows the code number, such as 10040*. These are called starred procedures, and they will be discussed later in detail.

As described above, normal, uncomplicated follow-up care is included in the Surgical Package. However, there are times you may want to report or denote (with a code) that your physician saw the patient for follow up. **CPT** recommends that you use the 99024 code to report these visits. The 99024 code, found at the end of the Medicine Section, is described as follows:

99024 Postoperative follow-up visit, included in global service

Since the code description says that postoperative care is included in the global service, it makes sense that the "charge" associated with this service is $0.

For the first time in the 2002 version of **CPT**, the Surgical Package described by the AMA closely resembles the surgical package described by the Center for Medicare and Medicaid Services (formerly known as the Health Care Financing Administration or HCFA). Let's take a look at the two Surgical Packages so you can their similarities.

MEDICARE SURGICAL PACKAGE

1. **Medicare Pre-Op**: This includes the history, physical, and medical decision-making that occurs before the surgery (as soon as the day before surgery), whether in the form of an office/outpatient visit, hospital admission, ER visit, etc. It includes hospital admission or office/outpatient or another visit that occurs before the surgery, but it does not include the consultation or new patient office visit at which the decision to operate was made. Pre-op services will be reimbursed even if they occur within 24 hours of the surgery. The modifier -57 (Decision for Surgery) will sometimes need to be added to the Evaluation and Management code that is rendered before surgery to identify that the service was a pre-op service. (See Chapter 11 on Modifiers.) *NOTE: Some carriers stipulate that a certain number of days must pass between the history and physical (e.g., the E/M) and the surgery in order to bill separately for the visit plus the surgery.*

2. **Medicare Surgery**: This includes the operation itself; that is, services that are a normal and usual part of the surgical procedure. It also includes complications as long as they do not require a revisit to the operating room.

3. **Medicare Post-Op**: This includes services rendered to the patient following the surgery. It also includes all

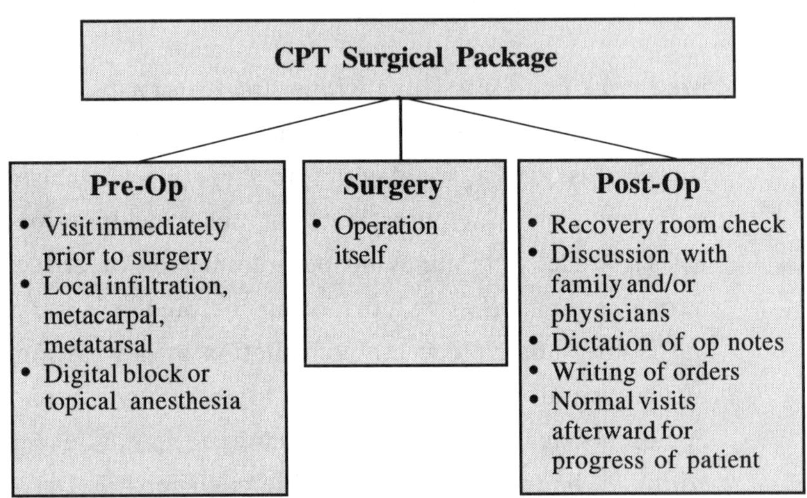
CPT Surgical Package
Pre-Op
• Visit immediately prior to surgery
• Local infiltration, metacarpal, metatarsal
• Digital block or topical anesthesia
Surgery
• Operation itself
Post-Op
• Recovery room check
• Discussion with family and/or physicians
• Dictation of op notes
• Writing of orders
• Normal visits afterward for progress of patient

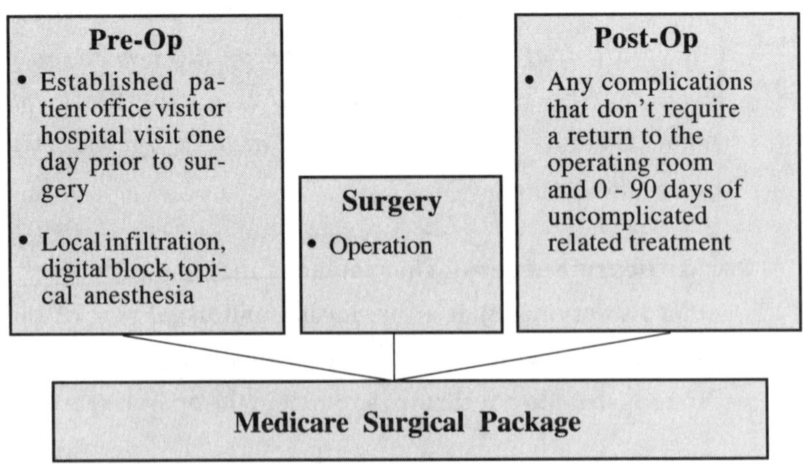
Pre-Op
• Established patient office visit or hospital visit one day prior to surgery
• Local infiltration, digital block, topical anesthesia
Surgery
• Operation
Post-Op
• Any complications that don't require a return to the operating room and 0 - 90 days of uncomplicated related treatment
Medicare Surgical Package

additional medical or surgical services that may be required because of complications, as long as they do not require the patient to return to the operating room. Depending upon the surgery, the number of post-op days can range from 0 to 90. Call or write your carrier for the most up-to-date list of **CPT** codes and their corresponding number of follow-up days. Use this list and make a note in your chart when you need to bill a patient for follow-up visits.

This concept of everything being included for one price is known to Medicare as the Global Fee Period. That is, payment is made for the whole nine yards (the blue plate special), whether it is used or not. If you need to indicate that not all of the Surgical Package (or Global Fee Period) applies, you will need to use the modifiers in the chapter on modifiers to indicate that.

The **CPT** Surgical Package includes the following:

1. **CPT Pre-Op**: The visit immediately prior to the surgery, occuring either on the date of the surgery or on the day prior to the surgery, so long as this was ***not*** the visit during which you decide to operate and the local infiltration, metacarpal/metatarsal or digital block or topical anesthesia (when used).

2. **CPT Surgery**: This includes the operation itself.

3. **CPT Post-Op**: This includes services rendered to the patient following the surgery, such as talking with other physicians related to the case or to family members, writing orders for the nurses relative to the patient's case, dictation on operative notes, checking on the patient in recovery and providing routine follow-up care. The **CPT** book does not list any time frames for follow-up care like Medicare does. Practically speaking, however, you would be well served to follow Medicare's guidelines for follow-up care as these are widely accepted by virtually every insurance carrier. Further, many physicians are inclined to offer more follow-up days (to patients) at no further charge than what is required by law. Adherence to Medicare's policy means that if the patient needed continued follow-up even after the maximum of 90 days, you could charge for it.

The major difference between the AMA's Surgical Package and the one adopted by Medicare, and hence, most carriers, is that the AMA has not placed a finite figure on the number of follow-up days that go with each surgery. Medicare has said that the number of follow-up days included with each surgery is from zero to ninety days (depending upon the surgery) and that services that occur after the ninetieth day are not part of the surgical package. NOTE: Some surgeries use less than ninety days to complete the Surgical Package because they are not as difficult to perform or to recover from. Your carrier can supply you with a listing of each procedure and the number of follow-up days considered part of the Surgical Package.

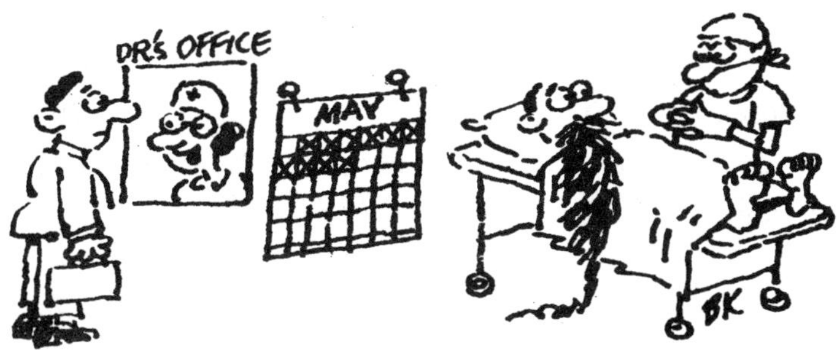

Medicare states that the Surgical Package follow-up can vary from zero through ninety days.

CPT Follow-up Care for Diagnostic Procedures

In the **CPT** guidelines you will find some information about what follow-up care is for diagnostic services. This will be discussed below.

Diagnostic procedures are those performed on a patient in order to find the problem. Diagnostic procedures include, but are not limited to, the following:

- ✓ Endoscopy
- ✓ Injection Procedures for Radiology
- ✓ Arthroscopy
- ✓ Laparoscopy

Follow-up care for diagnostic procedures includes only care related to the diagnostic procedure itself; it does *not* include care for the condition for which the procedure was initially performed. For example, if your physician performed an arthroscopy to diagnose a torn cartilage in a patient's knee, follow-up care for the procedure would include only care related to the arthroscopy, *not* care for the torn cartilage, unless the physician repaired the cartilage at the same setting (in which case, you would not use the code for "diagnostic" arthroscopy).

Another example is endoscopy. If your physician performed an endoscopy in order to get a biopsy, the **CPT** code would be the following:

43235 *Upper gastrointestinal endoscopy including esophagus, stomach, and either the duodenum and/or jejunum as appropriate; diagnostic, with or without collection of specimen(s) by brushing or washing (separate procedure)*

Follow-up care for this procedure only includes care associated with obtaining the biopsy, *not* care associated with the disease the patient may have, which, for the sake of our example, would not be treated at this time.

CPT continues the concept of follow-up care for diagnostic procedures by stating that care of conditions for which diagnostic procedures are performed is not included in the diagnostic service and may be listed separately (e.g., cancer).

Medicare Follow-up Care for Diagnostic Procedures

The Medicare policy on follow-up care for diagnostic procedures states, for endoscopic procedures, there will be no postoperative period for services performed through an existing body orifice. This is because no incision was made and therefore no "wound" would require follow-up. Services requiring an incision for the insertion of a scope (i.e., laparoscopy) will be subject to an appropriate time frame, between 0 and 90 days.

CPT Follow-up Care For Therapeutic Surgical Procedures

Therapeutic surgical procedures are performed to correct a problem. Their follow-up includes care that is usually part of the surgical service. For example, if it normally takes six weeks for a fracture to heal, follow-up care for a fracture reduction would be the amount of care that is normally part of that surgical procedure.

According to **CPT**, complications, exacerbations, or the occurrence of other diseases or injuries that require additional services are not part of the follow-up care that is related to the surgical service. Procedures and services provided to treat these unrelated problems should be reported separately, using the appropriate **CPT** codes.

If a patient begins to bleed following surgery and has to be returned to the operating room, the follow-up care that involves closing off the bleeders is not considered normal or uncomplicated and can be coded out separately. Some carriers may require the use of a modifier to indicate that the service performed was distinct and not part of the global Surgical Package. To illustrate this point to your carrier, you may consider using the modifier -78 (Return to the Operating Room for a Related Procedure During the Postoperative Period) or -79 (Unrelated Procedure or Service by the Same Physician During the Postoperative Period), depending on which more adequately describes the situation. See the Chapter on Modifiers for more information.

MEDICARE FOLLOW-UP CARE FOR THERAPEUTIC SURGICAL PROCEDURES

Follow-up care as part of the global fee concept for Medicare is between 0 and 90 days, depending on the surgery. Follow-up care is directly related to the service itself; it does not include services for a problem unrelated to the diagnosis for which the surgery was initially performed.

As you can see by comparing the **CPT** and Medicare follow-ups, the AMA does not define the number of days included in the Surgical Package, whereas Medicare does.

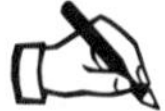

***Remember** that for Medicare, treatment for a complication which does not require the return to the operating room is included as part of the follow-up care.*

Materials Supplied by the Physician

According to this guideline, the physician who provides supplies for care of the patient over and above those usually included with the office visit or other services rendered may bill for those materials using the 99070 **CPT** code. Alternatively, National Codes may be used. These are found in the **HCPCS** non-**CPT** portion, where codes are featured for specific items provided by the physician, such as drugs, surgical trays, and casting supplies. There are many providers of durable medical equipment who have gotten national code assignments made for the supplies they sell/provide. If you cannot find a particular supply in the National Code book, check with your supplier to see if can tell you what number to use to code the supplies you purchase from them.

In general, Medicare's ruling on these materials (supplied by the physician) is that payment above and beyond the cost of the service provided in the office/outpatient setting will not be made except for drugs and certain supplies for specified procedures performed in the office/outpatient environment. CMS (Center for Medicare and Medicaid Services) has said that it will allow separate payment for some supplies provided on an "incident to" basis when they are furnished in a physician's office to treat a temporary condition (e.g., implantable catheter, see national code A4300, and surgical tray—see national code A4550). Separate payment is also made for splints (A4570), casts (A4580), slings (A4565), rib belts (A4572), special casting materials, light casts (A4590), pneumatic ankle control splints (L4350 - L4380).

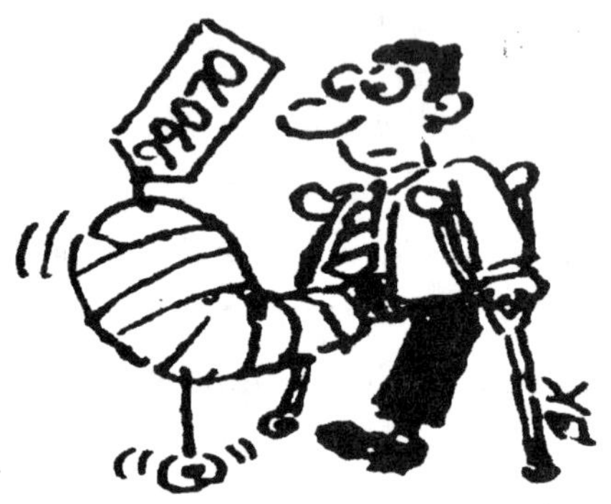

*According to **CPT**, supplies for patient care over and above those usually included with the office visit may be billed for using 99070 **CPT** code.*

Medicare will also allow you to be paid for surgical dressings if they are used to treat a patient's wound following a surgical procedure performed by the doctor. Primary surgical dressings are also covered as long as they are medically necessary. For more information on this as well as the number of follow-up days CMS has outlined for surgical services, consult the AMA's book entitled **Medicare RBRVS: A Physician's Guide** or the **Correct Coding Initiative**, (CCI) book. Copies of these book may be obtained by calling 1-800-443-7397 or by logging on to **www.medbooks.com**.

Finally, CMS has outlined procedures that when performed in the doctor's office will usually generate separate payment for supplies (usually surgical trays). However, in order to get paid for any of these procedures, you need to insure that you meet all of the following criteria:

1. The procedure can be done safely in the office, and that it is performed in the office less than 50% of the time.

2. The procedure requires specialized supplies that are not routinely used.

3. The procedure falls within the list of codes found in CMS's listing (CCI) or in the AMA's book, **Medicare RBRVS: A Physician's Guide**.

In other words, Medicare feels that the cost of most supplies is an integral part of the practice expense, and payment for these supplies should be included in the practice expense portion based on the relative value scale developed at Harvard.

Although the list of procedures is helpful, note that Medicare does not always specify for **which** supplies additional payment may be made; nor is it certain that Medicare's payment rate for these supplies will even cover their direct cost to the physician. It is Medicare's opinion that payment will partially offset the expense of the supplies and that the balance of the "savings" to the physician will be in time and travel saved by the convenience of performing the service at the office.

MULTIPLE PROCEDURES

Under the Multiple Procedures heading, **CPT** states that multiple procedures provided to the patient on the same day may be listed by separate code entries. An example would be a 4.0 cm layer closure performed on the feet (12042) and a complex repair of 2.5 cm performed on the cheeks (13131).

13131	*Repair, complex, forehead, cheeks, chin, mouth, neck, axillae, genitalia, hands and/or feet; 1.1 cm to 2.5 cm*
12042-51	*Layer closure of wounds of neck, hands, feet, and/or external genitalia; 2.6 cm to 7.5 cm*

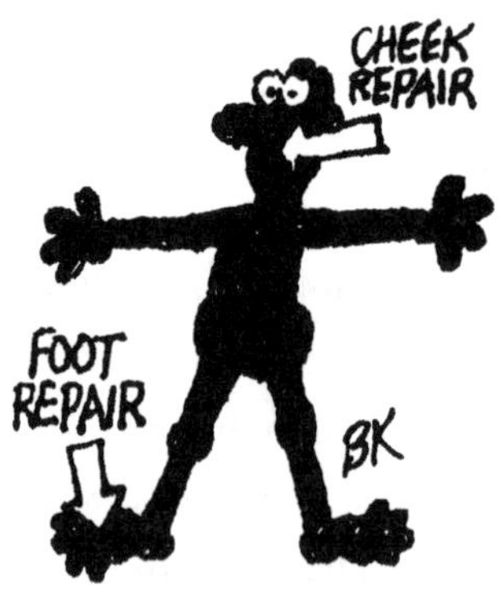

If multiple procedures are provided to the patient on the same day, it is okay to list the procedure performed by a separate code entry.

As you can see, it is appropriate to list as many procedures as were performed during a particular operative session, listing each procedure with its own price. The addition of modifier -51 to secondary (lesser) procedures is important in most circumstances and will be discussed in detail in the section on modifiers.

ADD-ON CODES

Add-on codes are those that allow the coder to "add-on" additional services to the main service. In other words, the services denoted with the plus sign are those that show additional procedures or services that are related to the original service.

Consider the following example.

*17000** *Destruction (e.g., laser surgery, electrosurgery, cryosurgery, chemosurgery, surgical curettement), all benign or premalignant lesions (e.g., actinic keratoses) other than skin tags or cutaneous vascular proliferative lesions; first lesion*

+17003 *second through 14 lesions, each (List separately in addition to code for first lesion)*

If you had a patient who had three lesions that you were destroying, you would use both codes, 17000* and 17003 in order to completely delineate your services. As you continue to learn about coding, it will be important to pay attention to the discussion of the HCFA 1500 claim form where the units column is discussed. It is in the units column that you will place the number of lesions (in this case one for the code 17000 and the remaining two others next to the code 17003) so that the carrier will understand how many lesions you actually destroyed. As the **CPT** book states in the guidelines of the Surgery Section, it is not necessary to add the modifier –51 for Multiple Procedures done at the same operative session (if you are using the add-on codes) as it is already understood that these services occurred at the same time.

Another example would be the following:

19125 *Excision of breast lesion identified by preoperative placement of radiological marker open; single lesion*

+19126 *each additional lesion separately identified by a preoperative radiological marker (List separately in addition to code for primary procedure)*

As was true in the aforementioned case with the 17000* and the 17003, this example of the excision of the breast lesion is another one in which you would use both codes (if you did two lesions) and would not need to use the Modifier –51 for Multiple Procedures performed at the same time. As the **CPT** book explains, add-on codes are exempt from the multiple procedure concept.

Most of the time, you will know that a code is an "add-on" code because you see words such as "each additional" or "list separately in addition to the code for the primary procedure" written as part of the description.

SEPARATE PROCEDURES

The concept of separate procedures is often confusing. It is probably best to describe separate procedures by giving an example.

Let's say your physician performed a hysterectomy on a patient that included a salpingo-oophorectomy. (Salpingo-oophorectomy is defined as "the surgical removal of a uterine tube and ovary.") The code for hysterectomy is 58150:

58150 *Total abdominal hysterectomy (corpus and cervix), with or without removal of tube(s), with or without removal of ovary(ies)*

The code for salpingo-oophorectomy is 58720:

58720 *Salpingo-oophorectomy, complete or partial, unilateral or bilateral (separate procedure)*

Note two things here:

1. The procedure for total hysterectomy includes removal of the tube(s) and ovary(ies).

2. The code for salpingo-oophorectomy, defined as surgical removal of the uterine tube(s) or ovary(ies), is followed by the words "separate procedure."

Note that salpingo-oophorectomy is included in the procedure described by the code 58150 for total hysterectomy. For this reason, it would be redundant (not necessary, and in fact, "double coding") to code for removal of the tube(s) and ovary(ies) using 58720 if you have already coded for a total hysterectomy using 58150. The salpingo-oophorectomy is listed as a "separate procedure" because it *can* be performed independently as its own unique procedure and not part of anything else, although it usually is performed as a component of the total hysterectomy.

The concept described above is worth repeating for emphasis. The words "separate procedure" mean you can bill for a given procedure if — and only if — it was performed alone, for a specific purpose, and independent of any other related service provided to the patient. If it was performed as a component of a larger procedure, and the description of the larger procedure includes the separate procedure, the separate procedure should not be listed.

Other examples of the separate procedure are some diagnostic arthroscopies, such as 29805:

hint

"Separate procedure" means the service can be billed if it was performed alone or not as a part of a larger "all inclusive" service.

29805 *Arthroscopy, shoulder, diagnostic, with or without synovial biopsy (separate procedure)*

Again, you can see that the words "separate procedure" follow the code description. This is because diagnostic arthroscopy can be performed by itself or as a component of a larger surgical therapeutic service, such as the 29819 code for surgical arthroscopy performed on the shoulder with removal of a loose foreign body.

CPT is very explicit on arthroscopies; it even points out that surgical arthroscopy includes diagnostic arthroscopy. Therefore, it would not be appropriate to bill for diagnostic arthroscopy unless the procedure had been performed by itself.

SUBSECTION INFORMATION

Important information can be found in notes at the beginning of the subsections, as well as sub-subsections of the Chapter on Surgery. For example, "notes" in the Musculoskeletal System subsection give information on casting and tell where to find appropriate codes for cast placement and replacement, graft procedures, fracture re-reductions, and suction irrigation. "Notes" in the Free Skin Grafts sub-subsection of the Integumentary System subsection help explain the coding used in that particular sub-subsection. Remember that notes in all of the sections serve as clues to optimal reimbursement and help reduce errors in coding.

Note also that when you see the inverted triangles (▸ ◂), the information listed between the two triangles is new or different for that year.

hint

When you see a paragraph or even a couple of lines that are not directly part of a code, read them! They point out important information that you need to know for insuring optimal reimbursement and reduced coding errors.

UNLISTED PROCEDURES AND SERVICES

Each subsection of Surgery features code numbers for unlisted procedures and services. These are to be used when you cannot find a description for a procedure or service your physician has performed. Effective in the **CPT** for 2002 is a new section called Category III codes in the **CPT** book. These are codes that can be used (and should be used) in place of the unlisted procedures (if applicable).

Let's say, for example, your doctor performed a procedure on a patient's orbit (part of the eye) for which you cannot find a **CPT** code. If the patient is not a Medicare patient (and thus is possibly not eligible for coding under National or Local codes), you can code the procedure by using 67599, a code number specifically for an unlisted procedure performed on the orbit of the eye. Remember also to check in the Category III codes found before the appendices in the back of the **CPT** book to see if any of them fit before choosing the unlisted procedure code.

Avoid unlisted procedure codes whenever possible, since their use delays the processing of your claim. In response to an unlisted procedure code, the data entry operator at the carrier's office is required to take several steps:

1. The operator will check to be sure no code is listed in **CPT** that could be used to describe the procedure your physician performed.

2. If such a code is found (because, for example, you were using an older version of **CPT** instead of the current book, which **does** contain the correct code), the operator will simply change your code and reimburse you on the correct number.

3. If no such code is found in the current version of **CPT,** the operator will either refer your claim to the supervisor for review or reimburse you on whatever procedure the operator feels comes closest to the one you described.

4. If you are submitting your claims electronically, use of an unlisted procedure code might get your claim automatically rejected.

The bottom line in any of these scenarios is that you will probably lose. Either your claim will be delayed while the processor looks for the appropriate code, or the supervisor will hold it up until she finds time to evaluate it and determine the amount that should be reimbursed.

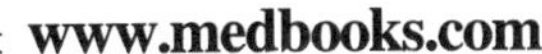

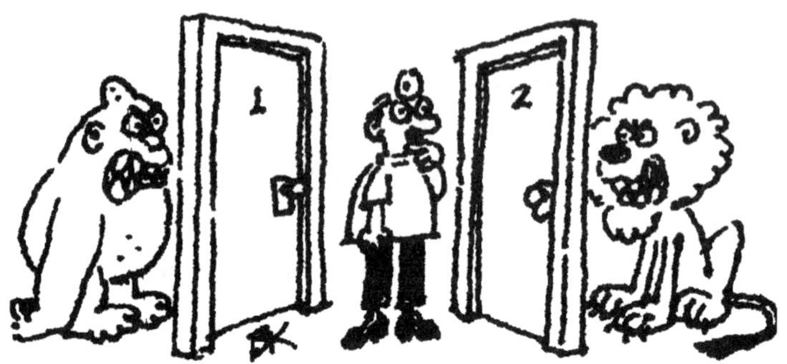

Try to avoid using unlisted procedures! You risk low reimbursements and slow claim processing. Either way, the fact of the matter is you will probably lose.

If you **must** use an unlisted procedure code, carefully and accurately describe the procedure your physician performed by adding a special report to clarify the procedure.

SPECIAL REPORTS

A special report is one submitted to the carrier to explain an unusual circumstance or procedure that varies from the norm. If the surgery was performed on an extremely overweight patient, for example, a special report may be in order. Surgery on such a patient is likely to take longer than the same type of surgery on a patient of normal weight, due to the special circumstance involved. I'm sure you can think of countless other examples that would warrant submission of a special report.

In submitting a special report, keep in mind the person with whom you are communicating. Picture yourself at the other end of receiving the claim form. What would make sense to you? A report filled with medical mumbo-jumbo you don't understand, or a clear, concise report explaining that the patient weighed 450 pounds, the operation was extremely difficult due to the patient's weight, and that the patient also had diabetes, which further complicated the surgery?

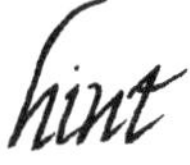

In writing a special report, you will need to use terminology that is easy to understand. Remember that the person on the other end is not a physician and that the operator is processing thousands of claims at a time. In order for yours to get the consideration it deserves, you need to make sure your special report is understandable.

What to Include in a Special Report

- Adequate definition or description of the procedure
- Time, effort, and equipment needed to perform the procedure
- Complexity of symptoms
- Final diagnosis
- Pertinent physical findings such as sizes, locations, and number of lesions
- Diagnostic and therapeutic services (including major surgical procedures) provided
- Concurrent (related or non-related) problems
- Follow-up care
- Pictures (if available) are also very helpful

Once again, the importance of keeping your special report simple enough for the average lay-person to understand cannot be overstressed.

MODIFIERS

The section on modifiers is probably one of the most exciting sections in **CPT**. Although modifiers will be discussed in greater detail in Chapter Eleven, it is important to mention here that those listed in the Surgery Section are appropriate to use with surgery codes.

Nine modifiers are listed in the Surgery Section. Every one of them can help you say something more about the procedure your physician performed.

Examples of modifiers will be given in Chapter Eleven. A complete list of those that apply to the Surgery Section can be found in the guidelines of that section in **CPT**.

STARRED (✱) PROCEDURES OR SERVICES

Starred procedures are only found in the Surgery Section of **CPT**. You will never find a starred procedure in any other section of the book.

A thorough understanding of starred procedures can generate additional revenue for your office. In some cases, starred procedures give you the flexibility of charging separately for pre-ops and post-ops, in addition to surgery.

Before we say more about starred procedures, it would be helpful for you to review the section in **CP"Teach"** that talks about the Surgical Package ("blue plate special"). Remember that the "Surgical Package" includes many things for the price of one.

In contrast to the Surgical Package, the concept of the starred procedure means that the Surgical Package does not apply and that you can code and bill for pre-op and post-op in addition to surgery when appropriate.

hint

Starred procedures mean the surgical package ***does not*** *apply.*

Suppose that two patients, Sally and Matthew, came to your physician's office, both with foreign substances in their bodies. Let's also suppose that Sally's foreign body is a splinter she is unable to remove, which is the size of a ball point pen head and Matthew was barefooted and stepped on a large piece of glass.

In examining the two patients, your physician decided that the appropriate therapy in both cases would be to remove the foreign body(ies) from each patient and that, in the case of one patient, suturing would be required.

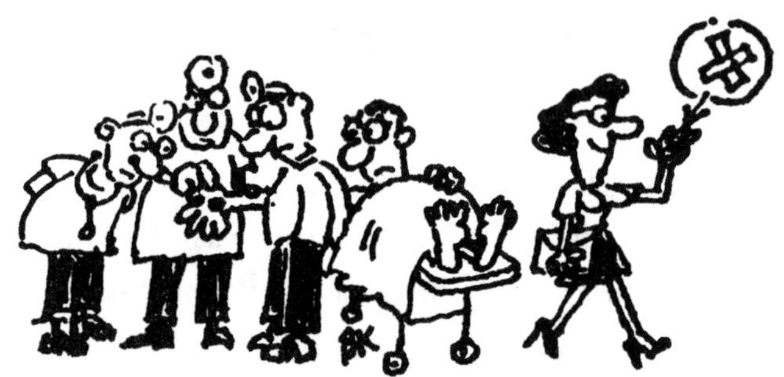

Even though the lesions may be the same kind for both patients, size may dictate the appropriate procedure(s) provided.

Services provided to Sally and Matthew could look like this:

Matthew's	*Sally's*
Pre-Op • Expanded problem-focused history • Expanded problem-focused exam • Straightforward decision-making	**Pre-Op** • Problem-focused history • Problem-focused exam • Straightforward decision-making
Surgery • Remove foreign body • Inject antibiotic • Supply antibiotic • Supply bandage • Suture	**Surgery** • Remove foreign body • Inject antibiotic • Supply antibiotic • Supply bandage
Post-Op • Reevaluate problem • Remove stitches • Interval history and exam • Discuss findings	**Post-Op** • Not required

As you can see by looking at these two patients and what was done for each, many of the services provided vary. If you examine the services closely, you will note that what caused the differences between the two pre-ops and post-ops depended for the most part on differences in size of the foreign bodies. That is, depending on how large the foreign body is or how infected it could become, the physician may do something different preoperatively and postoperatively in each case. In Matthew's case, the physician examined the affected body area and other related systems in order to make sure she had located each of the pieces of glass.

Because of the indefinite pre-ops and post-ops on some procedures, **CPT** follows such surgical procedures with a star. The star gives the coder the flexibility of both coding and charging separately for pre-ops and post-ops, in addition to the surgery itself.

If you were coding for the services rendered to Sally and Matthew, you would use the following numbers for each patient. (Let's assume that each is a new patient.)

Sally

99201 *Office or other outpatient visit for the evaluation and management of a new patient, which requires these three key components:*

- *a problem-focused history;*
- *a problem-focused examination; and*
- *straightforward medical decision-making.*

Counseling and/or coordination of care with other providers or agencies are provided consistent with the nature of the problem(s) and the patient's and/or family's needs.

Usually the presenting problem(s) are self-limited or minor. Physicians typically spend 10 minutes face-to-face with the patient and/or family.

*10120** *Incision and removal of foreign body, subcutaneous tissues; simple*

90788 *Intramuscular injection of antibiotic*

99070 *Supply of antibiotic (or better yet use appropriate "J" code from HCPCS Level II for supply)*

In contrast, let us look at Matthew's case to discover how the coding would be different.

Matthew

99202 *Office or other outpatient visit for the evaluation and management of a new patient, which requires these three key components:*

- *an expanded problem-focused history;*
- *an expanded problem-focused examination; and*
- *straightforward medical decision-making.*

Counseling and/or coordination of care with other providers or agencies are provided consistent with the nature of the problem(s) and the patient's and/or family's needs.

Usually the presenting problem(s) are self-limited or minor. Physicians typically spend 20 minutes face-to-face with the patient and/or family.

*10120** *Incision and removal of foreign body, subcutaneous tissues; simple*

90788 *Intramuscular injection of antibiotic*

99070 *Supply of antibiotic (use appropriate "J" code from HCPCS Level II for supply)*

99212 *Office or other outpatient visit for the evaluation and management of an established patient, which requires at least two of these three key components:*

- *a problem-focused history*
- *a problem-focused examination*
- *straightforward medical decision-making*

Counseling and/or coordination of care with other providers or agencies are provided consistent with the nature of the problem(s) and the patient's and/or family's needs.

Usually, the presenting problem(s) are self-limited or minor. Physicians typically spend 10 minutes face-to-face with the patient and/or family.

You may also consider using the 99058 code (found in the Medicine Section) with both of these cases for office services provided on an emergency basis.

As you might imagine, the total charge for all procedures will be different, even though charges per item will remain constant. The charge for the foreign body removal, the charge for the bandage and the charge for injection of the antibiotic will be the same for both Sally and Matthew.

If you refer to the Surgery Section guidelines in your **CPT** book, you will find information about starred procedures. For example, the book points out that certain relatively small procedures (such as the foreign body removal of which we just spoke) can involve variable pre-op and post-op services. You will also find other rules pertaining to starred procedures in the surgery guidelines of your **CPT** book. It is important for you to review each of these so that you completely understand the impact starred services can have on your reimbursement.

One final note before getting into a full-blown discussion about starred procedures. Some people say that the carriers do not recognize starred procedures. This is not completely true. Many carriers (e.g., Medicare) will argue that the Global Fee concept (with everything being included for one price) is the only concept that applies to all surgical procedures, starred or not. That's okay because in reality, the carriers and the AMA are basically saying the same thing. Remember that it is both the AMA and the CMS that give you permission to code separately for the service you rendered in which the decision to operate was made. This concept applies to all surgeries. In the case of the starred services, this would be the Evaluation and Management service that you provided before the surgery. If this service happened to occur on the same date as the surgery (as it would in a starred procedure situation), you would code for the E/M service (or pre-op as stated in the discussion of starred services in **CPT**) plus the surgery. In the case of starred services, it would be smart to employ the use of the modifier –57, Decision for Surgery, on the end of the code for the Evaluation and Management service. In the case of postoperative services, try consulting a book like the **Medicare**

RBRVS: A Resource Guide book that lists the number of follow-up days for each surgery. In this book you can see that the number of follow-up days for starred services is *usually* zero. As you know from the discussion on Global Fee Period, you are only required to provide postoperative follow-up for a set period of days (given to you by your carrier or found in a book like the one listed above). In general, as you will see by looking at the numbers of follow-up days associated with each surgical procedure, there are zero follow-up days for starred surgical procedures. This gives you the ability to code separately and bill for any and all services you provide following the surgery. Those starred procedures that do not have zero follow-up days behind them will warrant your consideration and observation and will require you to follow the rules of the specific carrier with which you are dealing.

Let us now take a look at the specific rules that the AMA gives for coding starred services. Most of these will make sense to you because you already have a clear understanding of Global Fee Period and what is and is not included in such a period.

Rules for Starred Procedures

Rule 1 says that a starred surgical service includes the surgical procedure only. When you bill, the price you indicate for the starred service includes only the charge for the actual surgery; it does **not** include charges for anything done preoperatively or postoperatively.

RULE 1

Surgical Procedure Only

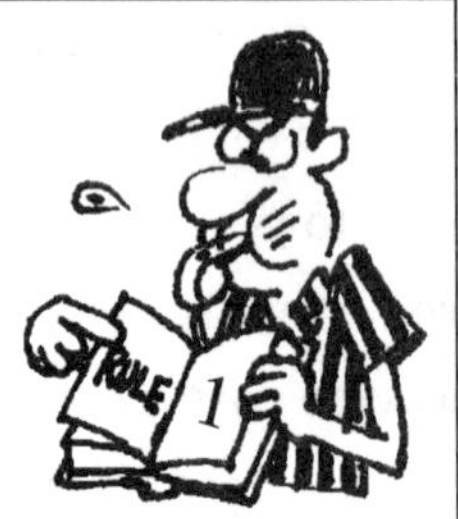

In the example we studied a few pages back, we showed that the surgery was listed by itself and that codes for the pre-op and post-op procedures (when they were performed) were listed separately. This rule makes sense when you consider the nature of starred services and how the pre-ops vary from patient to patient depending upon the severity of the case or the condition of the patient.

RULE 2

Use of Code 99025

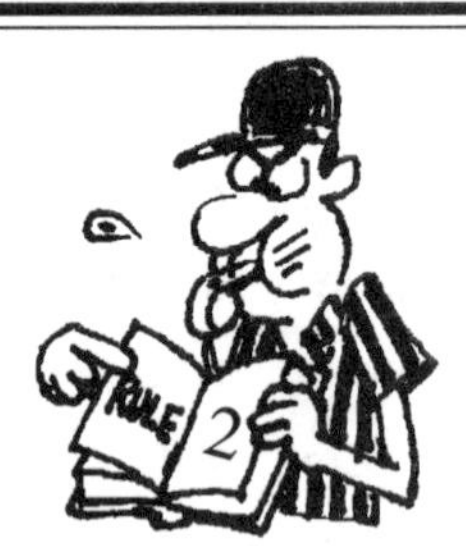

Rule 2 gives details about preoperative services. The paragraph under **Rule 2** discusses how to code for pre-op services in the event that a patient is new **and** the starred procedure is the only service provided. To better understand this rule, let's take another example. Consider the code 36415*.

36415 Collection of venous blood by venipuncture*

You would use this code to bill for a routine blood draw. Does it represent a surgical procedure? As you can see, this code begins with the number 3. According to the **CPT** numbering system, numbers that encompass the surgery codes are 1 through 6. Therefore, code 36415* **is** a surgery code, regardless of how you and I may feel about whether the procedure constitutes surgery. Because the code is surgical, the rules for the Surgery Section apply, and because the procedure is starred, the rules for starred procedures apply.

Let's say you are the coder for an OB/GYN office. You have a patient named Mary who has been coming to your office for years. Mary and her husband decide to have their blood tested for AIDS. (They want to have children but want to make sure that they are "AIDS" free before getting pregnant.) Because Mary's husband, Mark, has been relatively healthy all his life, he does not have his own physician. Mary recommends that Mark visit her OB/GYN office, suggesting that surely Mark can have his blood drawn there.

Because Mark is a "good sport," he agrees to visit the office of Mary's gynecologist. They go in together for the venipuncture.

Mary	***Mark***
blood draw 36415*	*blood draw* 36415*

Under the Surgery Section guidelines, you will see this kind of situation illustrated. The book says that when the patient is a new patient (which Mark obviously is to this office), and when the starred procedure constitutes the major service at that visit (which Mark's blood draw does), code 99025 is listed as an additional procedure code in lieu of the initial visit code.

Look at the end of the Medicine Section of your **CPT** book, under Special Services and Reports, and you will see the code 99025:

99025 *Initial (new patient) visit when the starred (*) surgical procedure constitutes major service at that visit*

As you can see, this is basically a code that helps to compensate you for the time and effort needed to open a chart on Mark. It is listed in addition to the code for the "surgery" or blood draw. Mark's bill, containing two codes, will appear as follows:

Mark

*36415** *Collection of venous blood by venipuncture*

99025 *Initial new patient visit when the starred (*) surgical service constitutes the major service at that visit*

From a practical standpoint, keep in mind that the likelihood that a carrier will recognize and pay on the code 99025 is slim. Further, keep in mind that the likelihood that you would not provide additional services that would qualify you to be able to code for another service (e.g., a regular E/M service) is also nil. However, the option for you to use the code 99025 is there (in the rare case that you do not provide anything else to the new patient while you provide a starred procedure).

RULE 2 ***Continued***

Starred Procedure is Major Service

Let's skip for a moment to other points made but not specifically spelled out under **Rule 2** concerning established patients. Although not specifically spelled out in the **CPT** book, consider what to do when a starred procedure is carried out on an established patient, like Mary, on whom no other significant/ identifiable services are performed (e.g., Mary does not plan to have her annual physical today). When the starred procedure is performed at the time of a follow-up (established patient) visit (such as Mary's visit), and when this starred procedure constitutes the major service at that visit, the visit itself of which there really was none, in this case, that included anything of significance (e.g., no E/M), is usually not listed as an additional service. You would only code for Mary's draw.

RULE 2 *Continued*

Starred Procedures with Other Significant, Identifiable Services

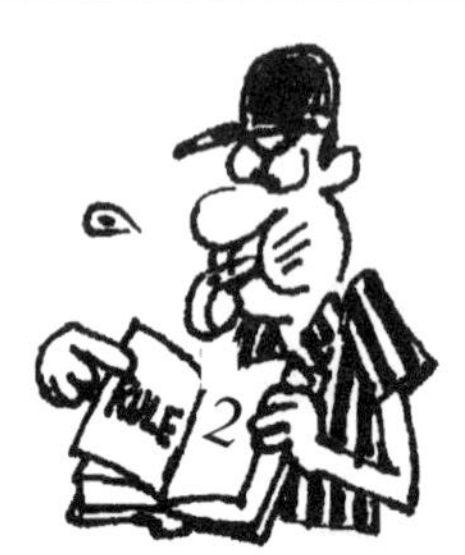

The inverse of that is also true. If the physician or nurse provided another service—such as taking Mary's blood pressure and weight at the same time as the blood draw, you could add the E/M code to the 36415* to show the procedures that are provided:

Mary

36415 Collection of venous blood by venipuncture*

99211-25 Office or other outpatient visit for the evaluation and management of an established patient, that may not require the presence of a physician.

Usually, the presenting problem(s) are minimal. Typically, 5 minutes are spent performing or supervising these services.

In cases like the blood draw examples, you may also want to use the code 99000 (found in the Medicine Section) that describes the handling of the specimen from a doctor's office to the lab. You will only have to use this if you actually did the work of handling and transfer to the lab.

Once again, if you have an Evaluation and Management service that you will code for in addition to the code for the starred service, remember, as recommended by the **CPT** book in these rules for starred procedures, to use the modifier –25 for Significant, Separately Identifiable E/M Service By The Same Physician On The Same Day Of The Procedure Or Other Service. In other words, you should always be looking for pre-op and post-op services (if applicable) to complete the Surgical Package.

As stated before and due to the Global Fee Package, generally no payment is made for a visit on the same day of the surgery unless a documented, separately identifiable service is furnished. For example, a visit during which the suturing of a scalp took place (starred service), as well as a full neurological exam for a patient with head trauma, would be coded with both the starred procedure code and the appropriate E/M code. Again, you would need to add the modifier -25 to the E/M service.

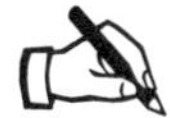

Remember, *when you use a starred code, you are coding only the surgery itself. Any pre- and/or post-op services also need to be coded.*

You need to complete the Surgical Package by coding for the pre-op and post-op separately.

Another example of starred services being performed with other major services is the following. Let's say that a patient came in for removal of a foreign body from her eye. The physician would perform a thorough eye examination to determine whether any other foreign bodies were present. This examination would constitute another "significant identifiable service." Thus, you would code not only for the foreign body removal (see 65205*), but also for the history, physical, and medical decision-making that occurred beforehand [see 92002 (an ophthalmology code since we are dealing with the eye) or the appropriate E/M code].

If you think about it, you will realize that no patient calls up to schedule this kind of service. A patient with a foreign body in her eye wants to be seen as soon as possible. Usually, this means you must fit the patient into your already-scheduled day. Because this is an office emergency, you can also use code 99058, "Office services provided on an emergency basis." (See Special Services and Reports in the Medicine Section for this code and others like it that may be added in special circumstances.)

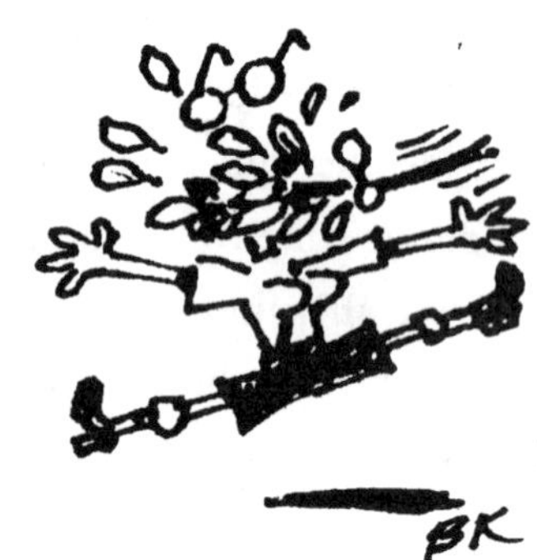

When a foreign body is in the patient's eye, the patient calls up and wants to be seen as soon as possible .

If special tools were used to remove the foreign body, you can consider coding and billing for use of the surgical tray with either the **CPT** code 99070 for supplies or the National Code A4550. **Remember:** The decision to use 99070 or A4550 for a patient depends on which carrier you are dealing with. Most carriers read both **CPT** (Level I) and HCPCS National (Level II) codes but prefer the specificity that the National Codes have for supplies.

Even though **CPT** gives you the flexibility of adding these services and supplies, not all carriers will pay for them. As stated previously, Medicare includes many supplies in the cost of the surgery because these supplies are viewed as part of the overall cost of performing the procedure. Check the procedure for which you are billing against the list given in the **Medicare RBRVS: A Physician's Guide** to determine whether this is a service for which supplies can be added.

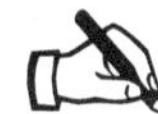

Remember also *that many non-Medicare carriers are using the Medicare National codes and will recognize the codes for supplies for their covered patients.*

Depending on the carrier, your coding for removal of a foreign body from the eye could look like this:

*65205** *Removal of foreign body, external eye; conjunctival superficial*

92002 *Ophthalmological services, medical examination and evaluation with initiation of diagnostic treatment program; intermediate, new patient*

99058 *Office services provided on an emergency basis*

99070 *Supply of surgical tray (or National Code A4550)*

As you can see, recognition of the star and its correct use can have a significant positive impact on the way you code, the total amount you bill and the revenues your office receives.

Another example of this rule would be excision of skin tags (11200*) at the same time as excision of a 0.5 cm benign lesion of the hands (11420). Notice here the two different and distinctly identifiable procedures.

In a case like this one, **Rule 2** under Starred Procedures in the Surgery Section guidelines would apply. As the rule states, other identifiable services or appropriate visits are listed in addition to the starred procedure.

You may ask at this point if it would be permissible to charge for a pre-op in this case because one of these procedures is starred and the other is not.

Both are surgical procedures (i.e., both begin with a number from 1 to 6). Since one (11420) is not a starred procedure, the rules for non-starred procedures would apply. This procedure would include either the **CPT** or Medicare Surgical Package, and it would not be appropriate (according to most carriers) for you to bill the office/ outpatient visit (or emergency or hospital visit) separately. In this case, the pre-op for code 11420 would serve also as the pre-op for code 11200*. It would not make sense to repeat the pre-op as part of code 11200* when it is already provided as a component of code 11420.

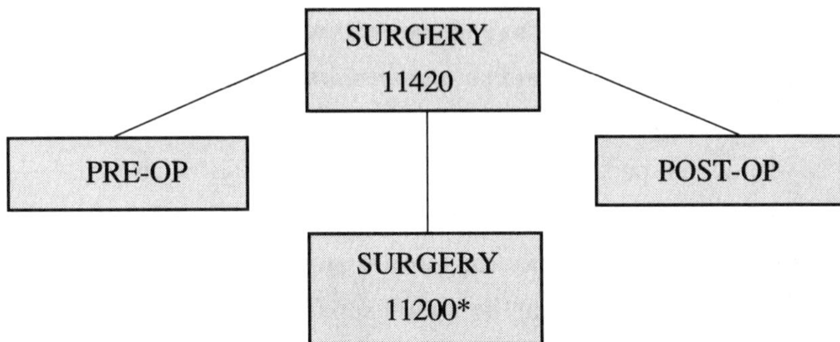

The coding for such an example would appear as follows:

11420	*Excision, benign lesion, including margins, except skin tag (unless listed elsewhere), scalp, neck, hands, feet, genitalia; excised diameter 0.5 cm or less*
11200-51*	*Removal of skin tags, multiple fibrocutaneous tags, any area; up to and including 15 lesions*

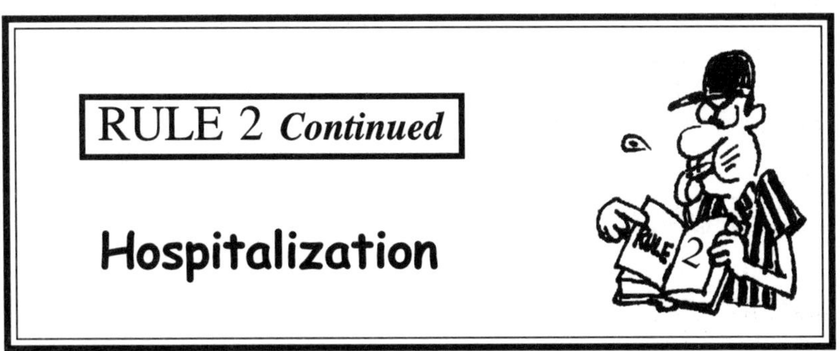

Rule 2 continues on to **say** that when a starred procedure requires hospitalization, you can list the appropriate hospital visit (or pre-op) in addition to the starred procedure. It is also appropriate to list codes for any follow-up care. This would be consistent with what both

the AMA and Medicare say about follow-up care and what is or is not part of the Surgical Package or Global Fee Period. Remember: both AMA and Medicare agree that the follow-up that is "covered" as part of the Surgical Package is that which is normally part of the Surgical Package. Complications that require a revisit to the operating room are not part of the normal Global Fee Period and can be coded separately. If you had to go to the hospital for a minor surgical procedure, such as a starred procedure, this could be considered a complication enough to warrant your coding the E/M codes for hospital...even for Medicare. If you are ever in doubt, please check with your carrier. Also, remember that most starred procedures have zero follow-up days associated with them, and therefore, visits following these surgeries are code-able.

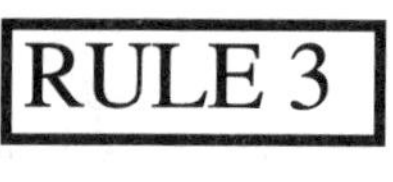

Postoperative Care

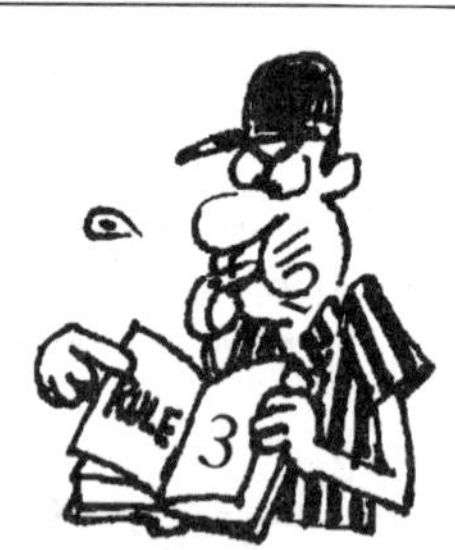

Rule 3 states that "all postoperative care is added on a service-by-service basis." If the follow-up care never occurs, naturally it cannot be added. If, however, two or three follow-up visits related to the original treatment occur, each can be added using the correct Evaluation and Management code for the visit.

RULE 4

Complications

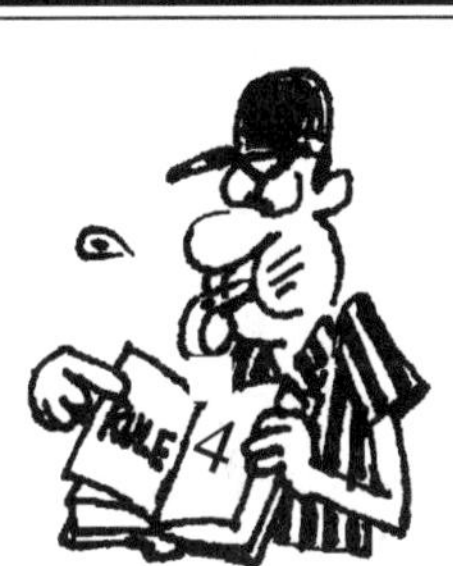

Last but not least, **CPT** specifies that complications occurring as part of the starred surgical service are added on a service-by-service basis. You might consider this statement self-evident, since you already know that any follow-up care for a starred procedure is added on a service-by-service basis and that many complications can occur during the follow-up period. **CPT** is saying that, if additional surgery is required (any procedure beginning with 1 through 6), this procedure can be added on a service-by-service basis; they may not be included with the regular office visit (or as part of the normal follow-up). This is also consistent with the Medicare policy that states that follow-up care included with the Surgical Package is that care which is between 0 through 90 days and which may include complications as long as the patient does not have to return to the operating room. If an additional procedure is required that is either unrelated to the first or requires a revisit to the operating room, it is code-able.

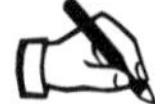

Remember: *Although Medicare realizes that starred services are minor procedures, a follow-up period of greater than 0 days may have been assigned to some of these services. Check before you bill for postoperative services on starred procedures for a Medicare patient.*

SURGICAL DESTRUCTION

The **CPT** book explains under this guideline that surgical destruction is part of the surgical procedure itself and is not ordinarily listed separately.

An example of this would be the lysis of adhesions in an intra-abdominal surgery. According to the **CPT** book, the surgical destruction of these lesions is included with the global surgery and is not normally listed separately.

If the surgical destruction substantially alters the management of the problem or condition, an exception to this rule applies and separate code numbers are provided for your use in the **CPT** book. You will look for these special circumstances codes in the sections within which you are coding.

Most of the Surgery Section is self-explanatory if you read all of the "notes" that apply to a particular subsection. There are, however, some sections that need to be reviewed, since coders in general have a very difficult time with them.

INTEGUMENTARY SYSTEM

In the Integumentary System, you will notice that there are many codes for which a measurement is necessary. In other words, in order to code for a removal of a lesion (benign or malignant), it is important that the coder know the size of the lesion.

Many coders rely on the lab (pathology) report to get the size of the lesion before coding. This is not always the best idea. Many times the size of the lesion has decreased after the specimen is obtained and the pathologist gets the specimen to measure it. The codes are often separated by 0.1 cm and it is important to make sure that the size of the defect, as well as the size of the specimen, are recorded before the specimen is sent to the lab.

An example of this would be the 11400 code that reads as follows:

11400 *Excision, benign lesion including margins, except skin tag (unless listed elsewhere), trunk, arms or legs; excised diameter 0.5 cm or less*

Notice that if the lesion diameter is greater than 0.5 cm, then the next code is employed.

You will choose a code for getting rid of a lesion based on several factors. These include:

1. How you got rid of the lesion (e.g., paring, shaving, debridement, etc.);

2. Whether the lesion was benign or malignant;

3. The location of the lesion.

Once you have decided the method, the pathology, and the location, you can choose the appropriate code(s) found in the Integumentary System.

Keep in mind that it is *not* to your financial benefit to code all lesions as if they were benign. Many coders feel that since they want to bill the patient and the carrier at the time of the service that it is just easier to bill everyone under the Excision-Benign Lesions subsection. Doing this will not only be incorrect at times (e.g., some patients will have malignant lesions), but it will also render a lower reimbursable amount for your office, resulting in a loss of revenue. In essence, just hold your horses. Tell the patient you have to see the results of the pathology report before you can bill him/her. If you must, collect some form of payment at the time of the visit with the explanation that there may be additional charges forthcoming.

The parameters for coding lesion removal changed somewhat in 2003 and became a little more specific. If you will look at the notes surrounding the excision of benign lesions, the book states that the physician needs to code for the diameter (the straight line that passes through the center) of the actual lesion plus the margins that the physician feels are conservative enough (yet adequate enough) to completely excise the lesion. This diameter measurement can be made through the center of the lesion in any direction (e.g., the diameter does not have to go from north to south for instance) and should be made such that it captures the maximum length of the lesion. The measurement of the diameter should be made before the lesion is actually excised from the skin so that the actual measurement can be as accurate as possible (e.g., once the lesion is excised, it may measure smaller than it would have before it was excised). Keep in mind that since the lesion diameter is actually the distance through the center of the lesion, it will be the same no matter what configuration the actual lesion is. For example, if the lesion itself looks like a leaf with edges that are not perfectly rounded, the diameter will be that distance through the longest portion of the lesion PLUS the margins necessary to completely remove the lesion.

Last but not least, remember that the codes listed for excision of lesions also include simple repair. If, however, you perform more than a simple repair (i.e., intermediate, which would include a layer closure of the subcutaneous and the superficial non-muscle fascia in addition to the epidermal and dermal (skin) closure or comprehensive which includes more than a layer closure) then the size of the lesion itself may be one thing and the size of the defect you repair may be something else. The significance of all of this to you is that you must make sure that you code accordingly because your reimbursement could be impacted.

Let's take an example. Suppose someone comes into your office for the removal of a benign lesion of 1.1 cm on his face (see 11442). Because of the location, kind, and depth of the lesion into the skin, a complex repair is needed. The size of the defect in our example is 1.1 cm. You would need to make sure you chose the code that went with that repair—in our example, since the repair was "complex" the code for repair would be code 13131.

A picture of a section of skin shows the different layers that you have from the outermost part (the part you can actually touch) all the way down to the bone. Understanding that the skin is composed of these different layers and what these layers are should help you in coding repairs.

It is important that coders be familiar with the three types of repairs found in the **CPT** book: Simple Repair, Intermediate Repair, and Complex Repair.

Simple Repair

Simple Repair is used when the wound is superficial and involves only the skin (epidermis or dermis) or the subcutaneous tissues. It does not include any involvement of the deeper tissues such as the fascia or muscle. Simple repairs include local anesthesia and chemical or electrocauterization of wounds not closed.

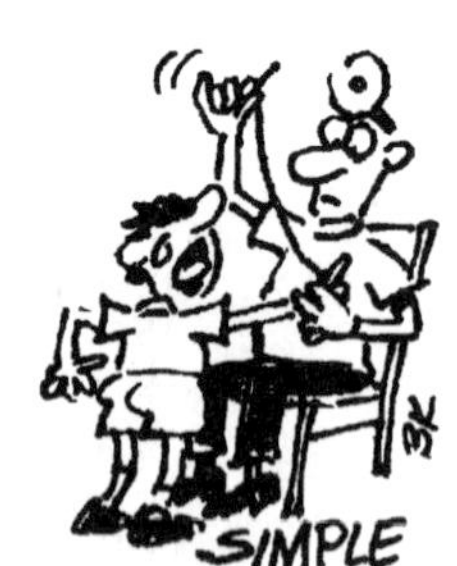

A simple repair requires one-layer closure

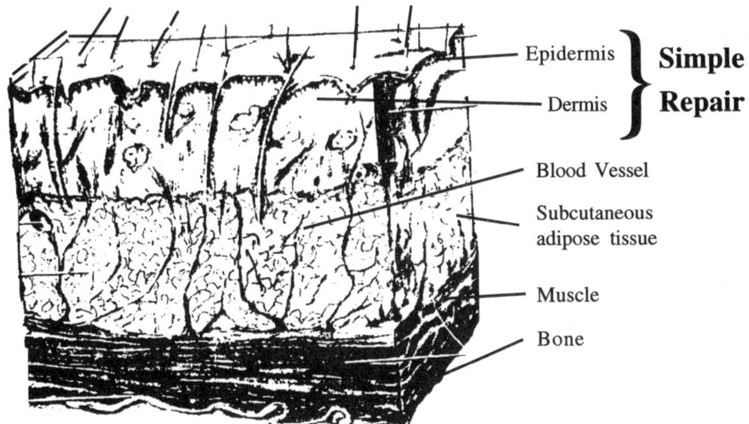

Intermediate Repair

Intermediate Repair includes a layer closure of one or more of the deeper layer subcutaneous tissues or superficial (non-muscle) fascia. The epidermis and/or dermis, the subcutaneous tissues, and the fascia are all involved. An intermediate repair is the kind of repair in which at least one of the layers requires a separate closure — or it could include a closure of a wound that has been contaminated and cleaned (if it is a single layer) or one that required removal of particular matter. See graphic below.

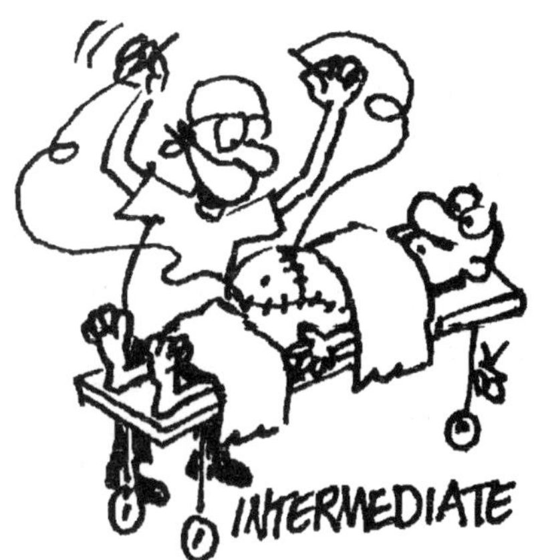

An intermediate repair includes a layer closure.

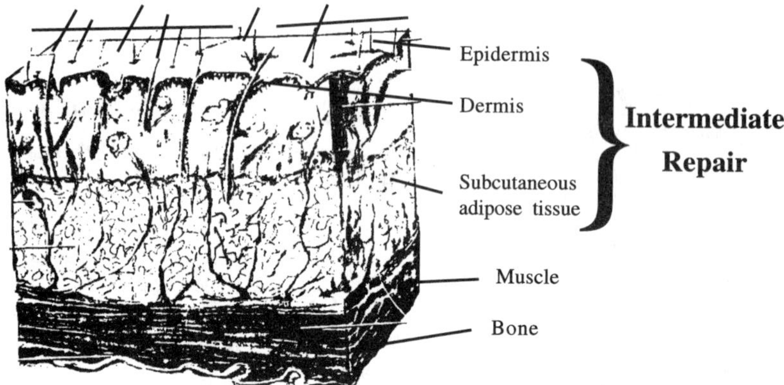

Complex Repair

Complex Repair is similar to a plastic (reconstructive) repair. It can be done for cosmetic reasons and includes such things as complicated wound closures, skin grafts, or an unusual and time-consuming technique or repair that helps in obtaining the maximum functional and cosmetic result: complex repair involves more than just a layered closure. A complex repair may include the creation of the defect. Examples of complex repairs may include scar revision or repairs of traumatic lacerations like dog bites or glass tears.

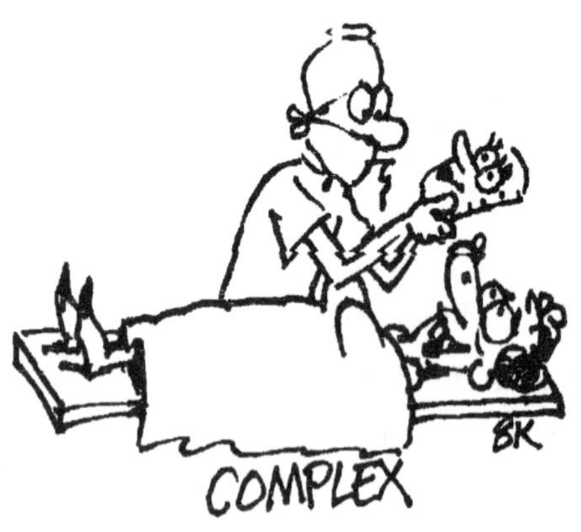

Complex repair is similar to a plastic repair.

Sometimes a complex repair includes the creation of the defect (for example, cutting away jagged parts to make a smooth finish) and the necessary preparation for repairs (e.g., excision of a tear requiring complex closure) or the debridement and repair of complicated lacerations or avulsions.

In the next section, we will discuss the rules for repairs and how they apply to your everyday coding.

RULES FOR REPAIRS

In coding for a repair, **CPT** lists several rules.

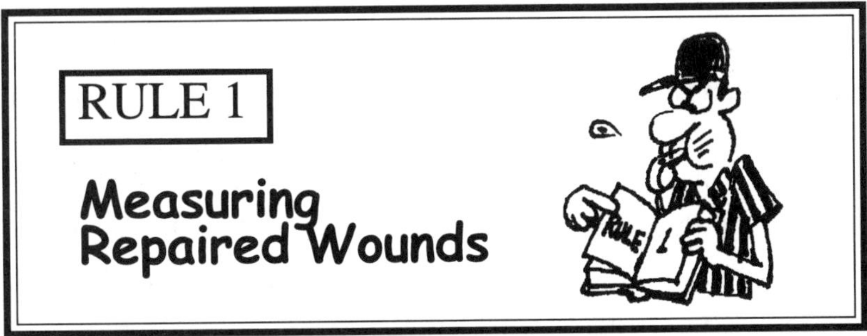

The first rule is that the repair(s) should be measured and recorded in centimeters. Keep in mind that in the United States we are used to measuring everything in inches. In **CPT** coding, however, it is imperative that the repair be measured in centimeters. Many people want to measure in millimeters and some even want to measure in inches. This is inappropriate, as the descriptions of the repairs in **CPT** are given in centimeters.

RULE 2

Multiple Wounds

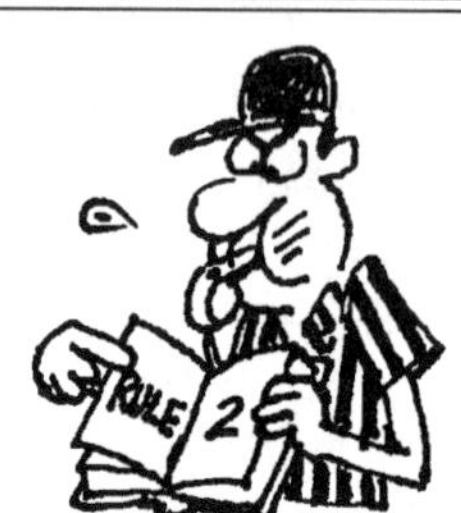

The next rule tells the coder that the repaired wounds, whether curved, angular, or stellate, should be added together and reported as a single item if they are of the same type. Simply put, you would add together all simple, add together all intermediates and add together all complex repairs. **CPT** says that in order to add together the lengths of repairs in the same classification, the repairs must also be in the same location given in the description of the code. To illustrate this, let's take an example.

In looking at code 12001*, one can see that the locations described for this simple repair are the scalp, neck, external genitalia, trunk, and/or extremities (including hands and feet). The size of the repair is 2.5 cm or less.

In comparing this procedure code to the 12011*, which is also a code for a simple repair, you can see that the locations described here include the face, ears, eyelids, nose, lips and/or mucous membranes. The size of the repair is also 2.5 cm or less.

In comparing the 12001 code with the 12011*, one can see that it would not be correct to add together a simple repair of the face with a simple repair of the neck. Each one would need its own separate code.*

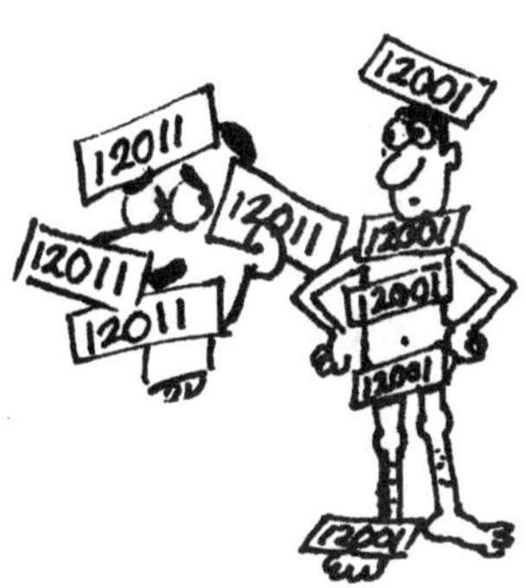

As you can see, it would not be correct to add together a simple repair of the face with a simple repair of the neck. Each one of these would need it's own separate code.

The next part of this second rule tells the coder that when more than one classification of wounds is repaired, (let's say a simple repair and a complex one), the modifier -51 for Multiple Services should be added to the lesser of the two procedures.

RULE 3

Decontamination and/or Debridement

Debridement or decontamination is part of the global service. This could involve freeing contaminated substances or the removal of foreign material and devitalized or contaminated tissue near a lesion to expose the surrounding healthy tissue. Decontamination and/or debridement would be coded and billed for separately only in these cases:

1. If you had to clean the wound for an extended period of time;

2. When an above average amount of the tissue is debrided or decontaminated;

3. When you debride the tissue and get all of the dead or contaminated tissue away and then wait until later to do the closure.

All three situations described above are fairly unusual and would, therefore, be reportable in addition to any code you may use for the repair(s).

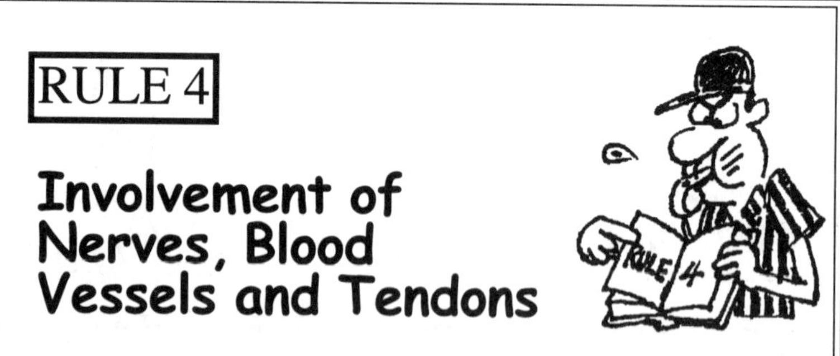

RULE 4
Involvement of Nerves, Blood Vessels and Tendons
RULE 4

When any nerve, blood vessel, or tendon is repaired, the appropriate code (found in the subsection, i.e., Nervous, Cardiovascular or Musculoskeletal) for such a repair of these structures should be reported instead of the code for the integumentary (skin) closure.

For example, in the repair of a cardiac wound (33300), repair of the integumentary is included in repair of the wound, and a separate code for repair (closing) of the skin is not needed since the repair itself is not considered to be a “complex” (as defined earlier) *type of repair*. Please keep in mind that we are not trying to minimize the fact that repairing a cardiac wound is not hard; what we are saying is that the *type of repair* (when we consider the simple, intermediate and complex types as defined in the **CPT** book) is not a complex repair.

There is one exception to the rule of not coding for an additional repair for the skin. When the physician, in addition to repairing the nerve, tendon, or vessel, also performs a *complex repair* on the patient as defined in **CPT** as a complex repair, to close the wound, the *complex repair* is not included as part of the larger procedure (repair of the nerve, tendon or vessel). The complex repair is reported separately.

Since the additional code for the *complex repair* is reported, you would need to add the modifier -51 to the secondary procedure(s) code(s), which indicates multiple services on the same day. Simple ligation of a vessel is also considered a normal part of the wound closure and is included with the code number selected for the closure.

Exploration of the nerves, blood vessels, or tendons exposed in an open wound, as long as the exploration is simple in nature, is also considered part of the essential treatment of the wound. Exploration of these structures during wound closure is essential. It will guarantee that no damage to the structures occurred during the wound treatment.

The only time that exploration of the nerves, blood vessels, and tendons is not included with the wound treatment as a procedure is when the exploration requires extensive dissection. In a case in which this is required, an additional procedure code can be listed in addition to the code for the closure. The **CPT** book has a special section that it has dedicated to the exploration and enlargement of wounds for trauma. See codes 20100 - 20103.

MUSCULOSKELETAL SYSTEM

You will notice if you look through this section of the **CPT** book that the codes fond here are arranged by body part from the head to the toes. Within each subsection (e.g., within the codes for the HEAD) you will find additional subdivisions which describe the kinds of services being rendered (e.g., incisions, excisions). Knowing this arrangement makes it very easy to find a code here; all you have to do is look under the body part, find it in the **CPT** book and then look under the kind of service you provided (e.g., incision, excision).

The subsection for the Musculoskeletal System features some items of major importance. The first of these is the placement of casts and strapping. Many coders, when coding for the initial or first-time cast placement when the doctor is trying to "treat" the bone, use the codes that are found between 29000 and 29799. This is incorrect! An example of one of these codes follows:

29425 Application of short leg cast (below knee to toes); walking or ambulatory type

In the notes under the Musculoskeletal System, **CPT** points out that services listed between 20000* and 28899 include the application and removal of the first cast or traction device. Using an additional code for the cast placement, or use of the codes in the 29000 series for the initial cast placement, would not be correct in most circumstances. (Remember: if you are using a special casting material that you have supplied (e.g., hexcelite), you may consider coding for that as a supply by using a HCPCS National Code.)

Reimbursement on codes in the 29000 series is based on the fact that these are codes for second-time placement of the cast or traction device or for the initial procedure when the doctor is only trying to stabilize or protect the bone. They do not include the "treatment" of the fracture; therefore, their dollar value is less than those found between the 20000* and the 28899 series.

Re-reduction of a fracture would be reported by placing a modifier -76 (Repeat Procedure, Same M.D.) on the end of the initial treatment code if the fracture was reduced by the same physician who did the first reduction. Modifier -77 (Repeat Procedure, Different M.D.) would be used if the fracture was reduced by someone other than the physician who did the first reduction. If you are unfamiliar with modifiers, please hold this thought until we get to the chapter on modifiers.

Here is an example of the use of a musculoskeletal code: Your patient fell down some stairs and suffered a fractured arm. Your doctor was called to the emergency room (at 8:00 p.m.) to fix the fracture. She determined that the fracture was a closed humeral shaft fracture and that it could be repaired without manipulation. She placed the cast and sent the patient home.

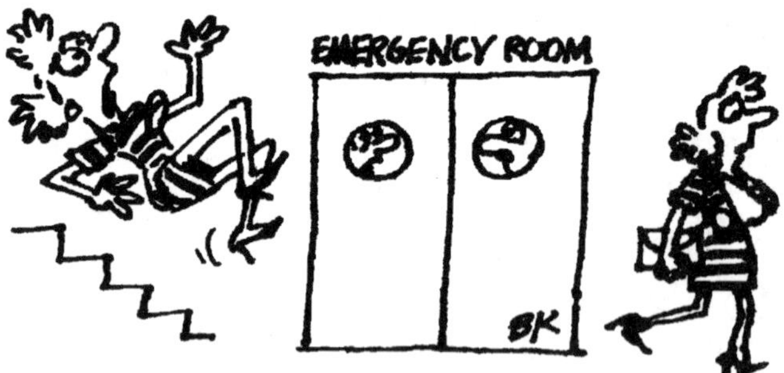

Your patient fell down some stairs and suffered a fractured arm. Your doctor was called to the emergency room at 8:00 p.m.

At first, you may be tempted to code separately for the different components that you see here. For example, your doctor is called to the emergency room to repair the fracture. Being called to the emergency room should make you think of one of two sets of codes.

The first could be the 99201 through 99215 series which describe Evaluation and Management levels of office/outpatient care and include a history, physical, and some sort of decision-making given in the outpatient/office; the second set of codes are the 99281 through 99285 series which also describe Evaluation and Management levels of service and are used when the physician is in an emergency department.

Since you will definitely need to code for the treatment of the fracture (a surgery code, beginning with the number 2), the Surgical Package will probably apply. Remember, you can only code E/M codes for Medicare if the E/M service constitutes the visit during which the decision to operate was made. Addition of the modifier -57, Decision for Surgery, added to the office/outpatient or emergency department code would be a good idea. However, you may still get a denial, as the history, exam, and decision-making may be considered your "pre-op." Watch for any denials like this on your explanation of benefits form. If you have gotten a denial on a claim that was properly coded (i.e., you used the modifier –57 on the end of the E/M code), you will need to resubmit the claim. If you were coding a non-Medicare claim and following the rules in the Surgery Section of the **CPT** book, coding for the office/outpatient or ER visit might be appropriate.

The next thing that should come to mind is the actual procedure your doctor provided to the patient. This would be the 24500 code which includes closed treatment of a humeral shaft fracture without manipulation. This code (as we just described) includes the application and removal of the first cast or traction device.

If you are coding strictly by **CPT** rules, remember that the "sequence" of events (what happened first, followed by what happened next) is not important here. You need to keep the procedures ordered from major to minor, and your carrier's computer can keep track of the rest.

If you were to look on the page in your **CPT** book that describes the application of casts and strapping (see the 29000 series), you would note that the 29000 series is for "replacement" procedures or instances when the physician needs to protect or stabilize the bone. Since your doctor *treated* the fracture, the use of the 29000 series of codes would not be correct.

According to Medicare rules and regulations, splints, casting supplies, and surgical dressings are separately payable under the reasonable charge payment methodology. (See section 1861 (s) (5) of the Omnibus Budget Reconciliation Act.)

If you placed a cast on a patient and ***no*** surgery was performed (e.g., you placed a cast on a sprained ankle), the **CPT** book tells you to code the appropriate Evaluation and Management code (e.g., Office/Outpatient or Emergency Department Services codes), once again remembering the modifier -57 plus the codes for the application of casts and strapping (see the 29000 series) and any supplies (that you provided).

He slipped on a banana peel and broke his cast! The "replacement" procedure is coded from the 29000 series of codes.

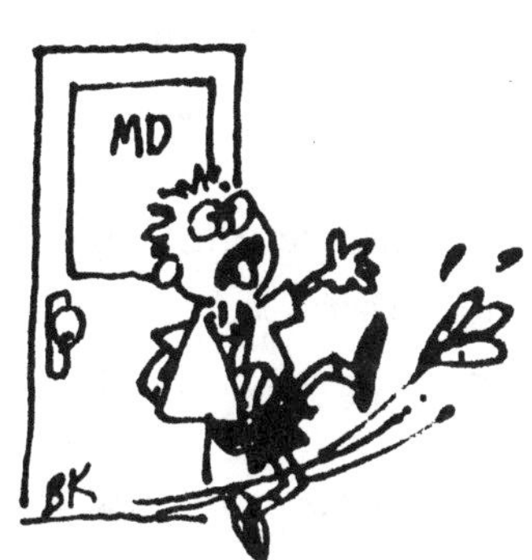

ENDOSCOPIES/ARTHROSCOPIES WITHIN THE MUSCULOSKELETAL SYSTEM

You will see that there is an entire section within the Musculoskeletal System that is dedicated to the coding of endoscopies and arthroscopies. These codes range from 29800 through 29999. Coding endoscopies and arthroscopies can be tricky, but the good news is their coding is the same throughout this **CPT** book. To illustrate this point, let's take a look at the following example:

29870 Arthroscopy, knee, diagnostic, with or without synovial biopsy (separate procedure)

As you can see, this service includes the procedure when it is done for diagnostic purposes and when the service may include a synovial biopsy. Suppose, however, that the surgeon discovered, once she was in, that the patient needed to have some loose bodies removed. What started out as a diagnostic procedure developed into a surgical one in which loose bodies were removed.

To code for this, the AMA says that you should not use the code for the diagnostic service; rather, you should employ the surgical code for this situation, which would be 29874.

> *29874* *Arthroscopy, knee, surgical; for removal of loose body on foreign body (e.g. osteochondritis dissecans fragmentation, chondral fragmentation)*

The fact that you would code for surgical service only (when the diagnostic one changed into the surgical one) is what was discussed when we talked about the concept of separate procedures. You will note when you look at the code for the diagnostic service that the words “separate procedure” follow the end of the description of the code. This clue, plus the fact that it makes sense that a diagnostic service could develop into a larger more comprehensive service once the patient is undergoing surgery should help in understanding that you would only code for the one service (in this example, the surgical one in which the loose bodies were removed) as opposed to both the diagnostic and surgical services.

You will see multiple instances of separate procedures throughout the Surgery Section. The concept of not coding both a diagnostic and therapeutic endoscopy or arthroscopy that is done on the same body part (i.e., when the diagnostic service turns into the surgical one) will be the same no matter what part of the Surgery Section you find it in.

RESPIRATORY SYSTEM

Once again, the arrangement of this subsection is from the top of the head, beginning with the nose and going downward to lungs and pleura. As you saw in other subsections of the Surgery Section listed above, the subdivisions of each body part (e.g., nose, accessory sinuses, larynx) are the same as you see in other subdivisions of Surgery, (e.g., incision, excision).

As you may already know, there are four major sinuses located in the head. These include the following:

a. Frontal Sinus: located on either side of the nose and on the front of the face at the forehead area.

b. Ethmoid Sinus: located in the ethmoid bone ("ethmos" is Greek for "sieve-like") next to the upper portion of the inner eye.

c. Sphenoidal Sinus: a wedge-shaped bone located next to the inner eye but below the ethmoid sinus.

d. Maxillary Sinus: located above the teeth [hence the name "maxillary" for the maxilla (teeth)] and on either side of the face.

As you can see from the picture below, each of these sinuses is separate from the others. That is, they do not interconnect and are not like rooms off of a main hallway. Just because you are in one of the sinuses does not mean that you can easily access the other(s). From a surgical standpoint, getting from one sinus to the other requires a significant amount of work. Because of this, the **CPT** book gives several alternatives for codes that describe the different sinuses. You will need to pay special attention to these differences

Paranasal Sinuses

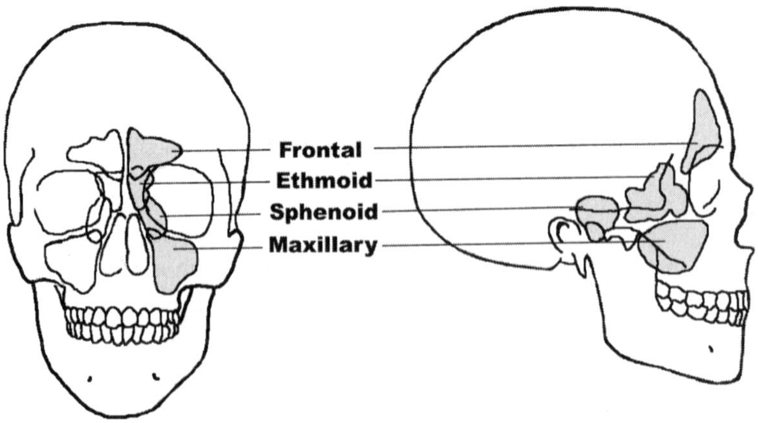

Frontal
Ethmoid
Sphenoid
Maxillary

in codes if you are using this section because the accuracy of your payments and reporting will depend upon your reading each description accurately.

To illustrate this concept, if you were to look at the **CPT** book under the Respiratory System, and in particular under Endoscopy in the Respiratory System, you would see many codes (31231 through 31294), each of which describes a different sinus and several different ways to get to that sinus. For example:

31050 *Sinusotomy, sphenoid, with or without biopsy*

versus

31070 *Sinusotomy frontal; external, simple (trephine operation)*

Another example of this is the following:

31233 *Nasal/sinus endoscopy, diagnostic with maxillary sinusoscopy (via inferior meatus or canine fossa puncture)*

as compared to

31235 *Nasal/sinus endoscopy, diagnostic with sphenoid sinusoscopy (via puncture of sphenoidal face or cannulation of ostium)*

As you can see by looking at the codes above, they not only describe different sinuses, they may also describe different approaches to get to those sinuses.

Many of the procedures that you will find in the Respiratory subsection will include codes that describe endoscopies (where an instrument is used to examine the interior of a cavity or, in these cases, the sinuses, trachea or bronchi or lungs and pleura) or incisions, destructions, or repairs. You will see that when an endoscopy is performed on one of the sinuses, you must be careful to read the different descriptions of the codes to make sure that the ones you choose describe the sinus you explored.

The procedures listed in this section are unilateral; they are done on one side. If they are not meant to be unilateral, the code description will tell you so. If you are using a code that does not say anything about being bilateral, and if you provide a service that is done on both sides, it will be important to make sure that you use a modifier (-50 for Bilateral Services) on the second side. We will discuss more on modifiers in Chapter 11.

Keep in mind that the codes 31231 through 31235 imply that you are inspecting the nose and sinuses listed above. You will be passing through the areas on the inside of the nose, the middle and superior meatus, the turbinates, and the sphenoethmoid recesses. Because you are passing through on your way to the sinuses, you will not try to separately code each of the inspections that you did along the way.

You will also see what we have already discussed about separate procedures here in the Respiratory System. If you refer to the codes for endoscopies, whether these are found under the accessory sinuses, the larynx, the trachea and bronchi, or the lungs and pleura, it is important to keep in mind that if a diagnostic service turns into a therapeutic service, there will be no need to code for the diagnostic service in addition to the therapeutic one if both are done on the same body part and same side of the body.

Let's take an example. Suppose you had a patient who needed to have an endoscopy on his nose. Once you went in, you discovered that the patient had some polyps in his nose and decided to remove them.

At first glance, you would be tempted to code the number for the diagnostic service, 31231, which describes the unilateral or bilateral nasal endoscopy. This would not be correct. Once you actually removed the polyps, you would need to use the code 31237.

For the sake of making the example a little more lively, let's say that when you were providing the service of removing the polyps, the patient began to bleed heavily, and you decided that you needed to control this bleeding. Note that the code you used above does not take the control of nasal hemorrhage into account. You would therefore need an additional code. Consider the following:

31237 *Nasal/sinus endoscopy, surgical; with biopsy, polypectomy or debridement (separate procedure)*

31238-51 Nasal/sinus endoscopy, surgical; with control of nasal hemorrhage

The point made here is that we need to code for all of the services that were provided except for the diagnostic portion that had already turned into the surgical service.

Coding for laryngoscopy, where you go in and examine the interior of the larynx, can fall into two categories:

a. Indirect laryngoscopy where a mirror is used to see the larynx and you don't see it directly, or

b. Direct laryngoscopy where a lighted scope is used to directly visualize the inside of the larynx.

Consider the following:

31505 Laryngoscopy, indirect; diagnostic (separate procedure)

as compared to

31515 Laryngoscopy, direct, with or without tracheoscopy; for aspiration

Notice that although both codes include the laryngoscope, the view of the anatomy (whether or not a mirror is used) is different.

Within some of the descriptions of codes in this subsection (codes 31505 through 31579), certain numbers include the use of an operating microscope as part of the procedure. Here are some examples:

31526 *Laryngoscopy, direct, with or without tracheoscopy; diagnostic, with operating microscope*

and

31561 *Laryngoscopy, direct, operative with arytenoidectomy; with operating microscope*

In addition to the examples listed above, there are other codes in this subsection (see codes 31531, 31536, 31541) that also include the use of the operating microscope. The point to keep in mind is that you have the available codes and descriptions to use when you provide services using tools like the operating microscope; you do not need to look for an additional code.

Last but not least is the subject of coding for bronchoscopic services. The main thing to keep in mind here is that procedures including bronchoscopy are considered to be bilateral. That is, when you look at one side of the lungs, you will also check the other. Because of the inherent bilateral nature of these codes, you will *not* need to use the modifier –50 to describe looking at both sides. For example, take a look at the following:

31622 Bronchoscopy (rigid or flexible); diagnostic, with or without cell washing (separate procedure)

This service includes the looking at all parts of the lungs, including the major lobar parts and the segmental bronchi.

It may seem hard for the new coder to know when a service is considered to be bilateral or inclusive of all parts. This will come with experience and is certainly not anything to sweat out here. When you are in doubt about something like this, you should ask your doctor if the procedure normally includes both sides. He/she will know the answer to this, and you will be able to code correctly.

Cardiovascular System

The most difficult part of this system to understand is the terminology; there are many words and/or equipment that the average person does not understand. In order to make our discussion of this system a little easier, let us review (alphabetically) some of the terms you will see in coding for services in this subsection.

- **Cardioverter:** a device that delivers a direct-current shock that restores the normal rhythm of the heart.
- **Defibrillator**: a device that also delivers an electric shock to the patient in an effort to counteract the small, involuntary

contraction of the single cardiac muscle cells that are either damaged or whose nerve supply is cut off and who act spontaneously on their own.

- **Fibrillation**: when individual muscle cells whose nerve supply is either damaged or cut off act on their own to cause stages of polarization and depolarization (similar to an on-off, on-off state); this sometimes causes the muscle to quiver or react intermittently in a chaotic manner, causing an irregular heart beat.

- **Lead**: The "connection" between the heart and the power source or pulse generator. In a dual chamber pacemaker, one lead comes from the atrium of the heart to the battery (pulse generator) and the other comes from the ventricle to the pulse generator. In a single chamber pacemaker, only one lead goes from the pulse generator to either the atrium or the ventricle. The leads are placed and positioned in the heart via the blood vessels (usually the veins). To do this, a procedure called a thoracotomy is performed on the patient. This procedure involves cutting the chest open in order to place the leads on the veins.

- **Pacemaker**: A device that is used to influence the rate at which certain things happen. In the case of a cardiac pacemaker, the device influences the rate at which the heart beats. The kinds of pacemakers seen most often in **CPT** include single chamber pacemakers and dual chamber pacemakers. Single chamber pacemakers have only one lead that is usually placed in the atrium or ventricle of the heart. A dual chamber pacemaker is one that has two leads where one is placed in the atrium and the other in the ventricle.

- **Pulse generator**: The power source (or battery) used by the pacemaker. It is usually fueled by lithium, a white metal. A pulse generator sends signals or pulses to the implanted electrodes either at a fixed pace or in a certain pattern. This makes the pacemaker work and helps the patient achieve a certain heartbeat.

Some of the nuances of the Cardiology subsection include placement and removal of the pulse generators used in the pacemakers. It makes sense that if the pulse generator is no longer working, the physician needs to remove it. It also makes sense that if the physician removes the pulse generator, he also has to replace the old one with a new one. If you examine the codes in this subsection, you will see that they only include one or the other; that is, they either describe the replacement or the removal of the generator but not both. Consider the following:

33212 *Insertion or replacement of pacemaker pulse generator only; single chamber, atrial or ventricular*

33233 *Removal of permanent pacemaker pulse generator*

If you provided both the placement and the removal of this device, you would need to make sure that you coded both numbers. The **CPT** book also tells you if you have to reposition the pacemaker electrode, pacing cardioverter-defibrillator electrode(s) or a left ventricular pacing electrode, you will need to use either 33215 or 33226 whichever is the more appropriate. This is a change from some prior versions of **CPT** where the repositioning or replacement of the device was included in with the insertion of the pulse generator.

It bears repeating to say that you must make sure that you completely read the description of the code before you use it. Services that are not described (e.g., radiological supervision and interpretation of the services, electrophysiologic evaluation of the defibrillators, electronic analysis and monitoring of the pacemakers or defibrillators) are all reportable using other codes. Generally, the other nonsurgical codes will be found in the Medicine Section of the **CPT** book, although they may be listed elsewhere.

More information on the particularities of each code number can be found in the book **Principles of CPT Coding**, written and published by the AMA.

Coronary Artery Bypass Services

These codes are only confusing if you do not understand that there are three different ways to report the various coronary artery bypass procedures.

These include use of the following:

a. venous grafts only;
b. arterial grafting using internal mammary or other arteries;
c. a combination of venous and arterial grafts.

Let us explore each one.

When venous grafts are used, there is only one series of codes to use (see 33510 through 33516), where the codes describe grafts done on veins (e.g., saphenous vein) from one through six or more coronary venous grafts. For example:

33510 *Coronary artery bypass, vein only; single coronary venous graft*

....

....

33516 *six or more coronary venous grafts*

Each of the codes between the codes 33510 and 33516 describes a different number of venous grafts.

When internal mammary or other arteries are used (e.g., internal mammary, gastroepiploic, epigastric, radial arteries and other arterial conduits that you get from other sites), you would use the codes found between 33533 and 33536.

A combination of venous and arterial grafts requires the use of the codes found between 33517 and 33530. It is important to mention here that when you use a combination of venous and arterial grafts, you will need to use two codes. The first of these will show that both the arteries and veins were used and will describe the number of venous grafts (see 33517 through 33523); and the second will show the number of arterial grafts performed (33533-33536). For example, let's look at the following:

33517 *Coronary artery bypass, using venous graft(s) and arterial graft(s); single vein graft (List separately in addition to the code for the arterial graft)*

33533 *Coronary artery bypass, using arterial graft(s); single arterial graft*

As you can see by reading the description of the first number, 33517, the book tells you that you need to select another number for the coding of the arterial graft. Just remember that you never report these codes alone; if you use one, you will also use the other.

Finally, it is understood by those who provide these services (and explained in **CPT**) that obtaining the graft from the saphenous vein is already included in the codes 33510 through 33523. If you need to improve the strength of the bypass graft of the lower extremity arteries, you will need to refer to the subsection that describes these techniques (see 35685 – 35686).

The last nuance of the Cardiovascular Section that bears discussion is that of the code 33530. In this code, you will see the following:

33530 *Re-operation, coronary artery bypass procedure or valve procedure, more than one month after original operation (List separately in addition to the code for arterial graft)*

Let's suppose that you performed a quadruple coronary bypass on a patient six weeks ago and, for some reason, you must redo the procedure. Your coding could look like the following:

33518 *Coronary artery bypass, using venous graft(s) and arterial graft(s); two venous grafts (List separately in addition to the code for arterial graft)*

33534 *Coronary artery bypass, using arterial graft(s); two coronary arterial grafts*

33530 *Re-operation, coronary artery bypass procedure or valve procedure, more than one month after original operation (List separately in addition to the code for primary procedure)*

Note that you will have to list all three codes to completely describe the fact that this surgery was a redo of one that you had performed six weeks ago. Each of these codes will have its own distinct price.

Digestive System

The Digestive System is arranged for the most part according to the passage of food from the mouth through the digestive process and out the anus. If you were food traveling through the Digestive System, you would pass structures which aid in digestion along the way. These structures are listed in the same order in **CPT** as the order in which they appear in the body. There are a few special nuances to be aware of in using this subsection. These will be discussed below. In general, make sure that you read any of the notes that you may find before, after or between codes. As always, those notes will give you special clues on the proper use of these codes.

Tonsillectomies and Adenoidectomies

All of the codes found within this subsection (see codes 42820-42836) are meant to be bilateral. That is, when you remove one tonsil or adenoid, you also remove the other. If you only remove something from one side, you will need to use the modifier –52 for Reduced Services on the end of the code you select. This modifier will be discussed in greater detail in the Chapter on Modifiers.

When you use the codes found here, it is especially important to make sure that you know the patient's age. Codes in this section (42820 through 42836) take age into account in the description of the code. You will also want to report whether or not you provided just the tonsillectomy or just the adenoidectomy or both the tonsillectomy AND the adenoidectomy. The descriptions take these different scenarios into account.

For example, suppose a ten-year old patient came into your office repeatedly complaining of pain in her throat. Upon examination, you suggest that this patient could benefit from having her tonsils removed. You remove the tonsils and code for the service in the following way.

42825 Tonsillectomy, primary or secondary; under age 12

hint

A primary procedure is when no prior tonsillectomy or adenoidectomy has been provided. A secondary procedure is when the service is done to remove leftover adenoidal tissue or tonsillar tissue or that which has regrown.

A few days later another patient comes in and receives a similar service (i.e., she has her tonsils out), but you recommend that she have her adenoids removed as well. You would code her services in the following way:

42820 Tonsillectomy and adenoidectomy; under age 12

Note that the codes here for tonsillectomy, adenoidectomy and services performed on the pharynx do not include controlling hemorrhage. If the patient experiences excessive bleeding (more than what is normally part of the operation), you can use the codes found between 42960 and 42999 to code for hemorrhage control.

Endoscopies

You will see codes for endoscopies (codes 43200 through 43272) like you have seen in the other surgery subsections we have already discussed. These codes will be used according to the same rules that we used for the other sections. Keep in mind that diagnostic services are used to view an abnormality inside the body (not visable to the naked eye). A therapeutic service is one in which the physician goes beyond the visualization of the internal structures and actually performs a service that is used to obtain a specimen, treat the condition, remove a foreign body or any other service like that. In other words, if the procedure starts off being diagnostic and ends up being used to "fix" a problem (therapeutic), you will only need to code the therapeutic services (e.g., 43202, 43204) and not the diagnostic ones. You will therefore see a lot of code descriptions for the diagnostic services within this subsection use the words "separate procedures". As you will recall from our earlier discussion of separate procedures, the only time we code for a "separate procedure" is when the service is done separately and independently of a larger, more global service.

Let's consider another point about coding for endoscopies within the Digestive System. Make sure that you code the appropriate code based upon *where* the service began. For instance, if you began the endoscopy in the esophagus, you would need to use the code found under the the description of the codes that lists the word "esophagus" as part of the verbiage. Likewise, if you began the endoscopy in the small intestine, you would need to select the endoscopy codes from the endoscopic subsection that talks about the intestines. If you were examining the rectum and sigmoid colon, you would use either the proctosigmoidoscopy codes (see 45300 - 45327) or the sigmoidoscopy codes (45330- 45345). Colonoscopy codes are reported with 45355 through 45387, and anoscopy codes are reported with 46600 through 46615.

Finally, you will see codes in the **CPT** book that refer to hernia repair (see codes 49491 through 49611). It is important to note that hernias are categorized in the following way:

a. **By type of hernia**: *inguinal* (into the inguinal canal), *lumbar* (in the lumbar region of the back), *femoral* (into the femoral canal), *incisional* or *ventral* (occurring at the site of a previously made incision on the abdominal wall), *epigastric* (through the linea alba above the navel), *umbilical* (protrusion of part of the intestine at the umbilicus or belly button), *spigelian* (abdominal hernia through the linea semilunaris), *omphalocele* (when a part of the intestine protrudes through a large defect in the abdominal wall at the umbilicus at birth).

b. **By method of repair**. A *reducible* hernia is one that can be corrected by manipulation by the physician. The hernia is able to move freely through the hernia opening. An *incarcerated* hernia (in whole or in part) is not able to move freely (e.g., it is incarcerated or "in jail") in the hernia sac and therefore cannot be manipulated by the physician. A *strangulated* hernia is one that is, as the name implies, strangled and constricted and where the blood supply to the area is affected.

c. **By previous hernia repair**: An *initial* treatment means that the hernia can be put back into its normal body cavity without surgery. You would code for the initial hernia treatment using an E/M code. A *recurrent* hernia treatment means that the hernia has already been (at some point in the past) surgically treated and placed back into its normal body cavity.

d. **By patient age.**

Use of mesh to repair the opening of the hernia is not coded separately unless you are coding for an incisional (ventral) repair. If you are providing an incisional or ventral repair, you need to make sure to code separately for the supply of the mesh if you provided it. Consider using the HCPCS National Codes for this supply.

URINARY SYSTEM SUBSECTION

Like other subsections within the Surgery Section, the Urinary System in **CPT** is arranged from top to bottom. That is, as you can see by the diagram, procedures done on kidneys are listed first, services on the ureters are next and so on.

In the Urinary System subsection (50010 through 53899), remember that some endoscopic services are listed so that all of the minor related functions do not have to be listed separately.

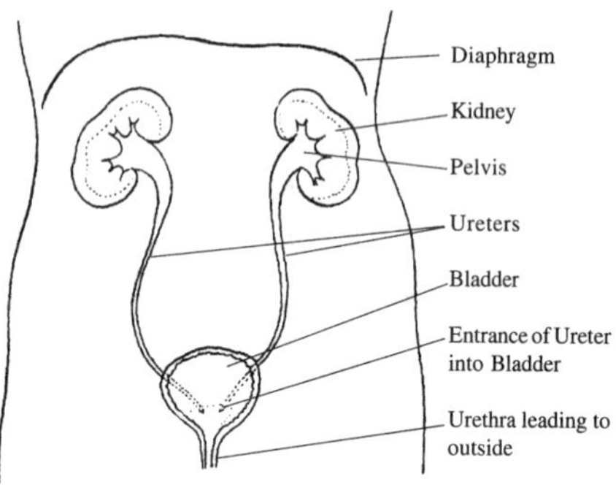

For example, let's say that you had a patient who received a non-contact laser coagulation of the prostate (see code 52647). This service would include (as stated in its description) the following:

a. control of postoperative bleeding;

b. vasectomy;

c. meatotomy;

d. cystourethroscopy;
e. urethral calibration and/or dilation;
f. internal urethrotomy.

In other words, you would not need to list all of these services out separately in addition to the code for the non-contact laser coagulation of the prostate.

As always, careful review of each of the descriptions you may employ is paramount before choosing a **CPT** code for your claim form.

You will see the words "separate procedure" listed after the minor related procedures (e.g., you will see the words separate procedures following the description for meatotomy-see code 53020). As you can see from looking at the description above, the meatotomy is part of the non-contact laser coagulation of the prostate. There may be instances, however, when the services that are considered an inherent part of the global services end up requiring enough extra time and effort to warrant their coding on an individual basis. When the secondary services that are already listed as part of the global services require significant additional time, or when the secondary services that you provide at the same time as the main service and at the same site are necessary to report, the secondary procedure may be further identified by addition of the modifier -22 for Unusual Services to the secondary procedure code.

The AMA gives the following example of this in its book, **Principles of CPT Coding**. Let's say that an urethrotomy was performed for a documented, preexisting stricture or bladder neck contracture prior to a transurethral resection of the prostate. If you were to look at the code for the transurethral resection of the prostate, you would see the following:

52601 *Transurethral electrosurgical resection of prostate, including control of postoperative bleeding, complete (vasectomy, meatotomy, cystourethroscopy, urethral calibration and/or dilation, and internal urethrotomy are included)*

As you can see, the urethrotomy is part of the global service as listed in code 52601. In this example, however, when the urethrotomy is performed for a documented, preexisting stricture or when it requires a significant amount of extra work to merit coding an extra code you would need to add the modifier –22 for Unusual Services to the end of the code for the urethrotomy (see code 53000). Although we will discuss more about the modifier –22 for Unusual Services in the Chapter on Modifiers, just make a note to yourself that you may need to submit a special report with this claim in order to get it paid.

As you will see in the Chapter on Medicine, the supply of drugs is not included in with the code for an injection with the exception of the codes and supplies listed under Immune Globulins, Vaccines, or Toxoids. You will see codes in this Urinary System Section (e.g., *52283 Cystourethroscopy, with steroid injection into stricture -*

Copyright AMA, 2002) that describe injections but that do not include the supply on any steroids (drugs). If you supply the drugs, you will need to code for them separately using the HCPCS National Codes for supplies.

Female Genital System

The codes covering the female genital system range from 56405 through 59899.

As we have seen throughout other subsections of the Surgery Section, the divisions of the female genital system are arranged from the northern part of the body going south. Also, within a particular subsection, you will see the headings for incisions, excisions, etc.

Once again, the terminology used in the **CPT** book within this subsection could use some explanation. The following words merit special consideration.

a. **Simple vulvectomy**. In this procedure, only the skin and superficial subcutaneous tissues are removed.

b. **Radical vulvectomy**. This procedure includes the removal of the skin and the deep subcutaneous tissues.

c. **Partial vulvectomy**. This service means that up to 80% of the vulvar tissue was removed.

d. **Complete vulvectomy**. This service indicates that more than 80% of the vulvar tissue was removed.

These words will be important to your coding and understanding of the codes 56620 through 56640. For example:

56620 *Vulvectomy simple; partial*

56625 *complete*

As you can see by looking at the codes above, combinations of the words defined above can exist within a given code. The 56620 describes the fact that only the skin and superficial subcutaneous tissues are removed on up to 80% of the vulvar tissues. The code 56625 describes the fact that the skin and subcutaneous tissues were removed on more than 80% of the vulvar tissues.

You will also see the word "non-obstetrical" used in some of the descriptions of the various codes (e.g., 56810 *Perineoplasty, repair of perineum, non-obstetrical* - Copyright AMA, 2002). When you see the word "non-obstetrical" in the description of a code, make sure to only use the code when it is not performed as part of an obstetric procedure (perineoplasty may already be considered part of the delivery of a newborn, for example, and would not warrant a separate code when used in the newborn situation).

The concept of bilateral services is once again seen in this subsection. For example, it is understood that when you perform a tubal ligation that you expect to ligate (or close) both of the tubes. You would not need to use the modifier for bilateral procedures when the description of the code already indicates the bilateral nature of the service. Most of the time, you can use common sense to decide whether or not a service would be bilateral. This should make it easier for you when you go to code; just ask yourself what the "normal" situation would be (e.g., it is "normal" that a person would want to have both tubes closed usually to prevent pregnancy as opposed to only having one closed)?

With regard to the insertion and fitting of devices such as a pessary, diaphragm, cervical cap or intrauterine device, keep in mind that none of the **CPT** codes include the supply of this equipment. If you provided such devices, you would need to go to the HCPCS National Codes (e.g., see A4560 for pessary, A4261 for cervical cap, etc.).

You will note that the codes for both the insertion of the pessary (57160*) and the codes for insertion of the intrauterine device (58300*) are both starred services. Keep in mind that they are also both considered to be "surgical" services, and the rules regarding surgeries/starred procedures apply. As we already know, when a starred service is performed, we need to look for the preoperative and postoperative portions of the surgery. In these cases, if a woman came into your office during her regular yearly visit and you decided to place a pessary into her, you would need to code the following:

*57160** *Fitting and insertion of pessary or other intravaginal support device*

992_ _-57 *To code for the appropriate office visit depending upon what else you did during that visit*

A4560 *Supply of the pessary*

Many people fear that Medicare does not view starred procedures like the AMA does. Remember that the AMA and Medicare (as of the 2002 version of **CPT**) are basically on the same page with reference to what constitutes the Surgical Package. Both agree that the visit that happens prior to the "surgery" (any code that starts off with a 1 through a 6), during which the physician decides to "operate," is code-able independently of (and in addition to) the code for the surgery. It is safe to use the -25 Significant, Separately Indentifiable E/M Service By The Same Physician On The Same Day Of The Othe Procedure Or Service), –57 modifier (Decision for Surgery) or, on the end of the Evaluation and Management code to remind the carrier that this service was not part of the Global Fee Period.

In Maternity Care and Delivery (59000 - 59899), under the Female Genital System subsection, the codes listed include services normally provided in uncomplicated maternity cases (antepartum care, the delivery itself, and normal, uncomplicated postpartum care).

Antepartum care includes the following:

- *Initial and subsequent history and physical exams;*
- *Recording of blood pressures and weights of the mom;*
- *Recording fetal heart tones;*
- *Routine chemical urinalysis;*
- *Monthly visits up to 28 weeks gestation;*
- *Biweekly visits from 28 weeks to 36 weeks gestation;*
- *Weekly visits until delivery.*

Any other visits or services provided that are not listed above (e.g., monitoring of the patient in a pre-term labor situation or hospital observation, etc.) and that occur during this time frame need to be coded separately.

Delivery includes the following:

- *Admission to the hospital;*
- *Admission history and physical exam;*
- *Management of uncomplicated labor*;
- *Vaginal delivery (with or without the episiotomy and with or without forceps) or cesarean delivery.*

Since many patients need to have their labor induced with Pitocin, it is considered to be an inclusive part of the total obstetrical package and it is not reported separately. Included in with this all-inclusive

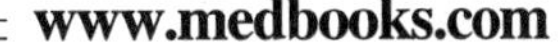

concept of total obstetrical care is the artificial rupture of membranes. Additionally, an episiotomy and forceps delivery are included if you provide the delivery. There is no need to code them out separately. Likewise, there is no need to subtract them using a Reduced Services modifier (see modifier –52) if you did not provide them. If you found yourself providing a vacuum extraction during a vaginal delivery, you could notify the carrier of this by using a diagnosis code that would describe this fact. There will not, however, be a separate **CPT** code for vacuum extraction as it is also considered part of the total package.

If you provided the total obstetrical care and delivered twins, the AMA says that you have options on how you could report this.

a. If the children were delivered vaginally, choose a code that most closely describes the care (see 59400 or 59610), and use the modifier –22 for Unusual Services, or

b. Use the 59400 or 59610 for the first twin and use the code 59409 or 59612 to report the vaginal delivery only of the second twin.

c. If one child was delivered vaginally and the other was delivered by cesarean section, you should report the code for the total obstetrical care with C-section (see 59510 or 59618) and the vaginal delivery, only code for the other child (see 59409 or 59612).

At any rate, how you should report these particular situations varies from carrier to carrier. Please check with your carrier to see what their policy is regarding this issue.

Medical problems that may complicate the patient's labor and delivery and may require additional resources, such as cardiac problems, toxemia, diabetes, and pre-term labor, should be identified by using the codes found in the Medicine or Evaluation and Management Section in addition to the codes for Maternity Care.

Postpartum care includes the following:

- Hospital visits following vaginal or cesarean delivery;
- Office visits following vaginal or cesarean delivery.

You will find that there are separate codes for maternity care and delivery for someone who has never had a C-section (see 59400 - 59430) and ones for the same kind of care on someone who has had a previous C-section (see 59510 through 59622). There is also a separate code for routine care for a C-section delivery (see 59510).

Services provided due to complications like pre-term labor or toxemia of pregnancy for example are NOT included in the "package" we just discussed. You will need to code for them separately, using either the Evaluation and Management codes, if the treatment is non-invasive, or the Surgery codes if the treatment is invasive (e.g., appendectomy during pregnancy).

USE OF CATEGORY III CODES IN MATERNITY CARE AND DELIVERY

In the 2002 version of the **CPT** book, there is an additional section toward the back of the book, near the appendices. This section includes Category III codes. Here you will find codes that are considered "temporary" codes. It is the purpose of this section to provide codes to physicians who may need them and for carriers to monitor the code usage to see if these codes need to be added to future versions of the **CPT** book or HCPCS National Codes. The Category III codes are alphanumeric codes but they are different from the HCPCS National Codes (that are also alphanumeric) in that the Category III codes have the alpha character following the number (e.g., 0001T, 0002T, etc.). You will notice that there is a code number in the Category III codes that can be used in the Maternity Care and Delivery section. It is the following:

0021T *Insertion of transcervical or transvaginal fetal oximetry sensor*

Feel free to use this code if you provide this service, but keep in mind that it may not be around in future years as the same number (i.e., it may not be around as the code 0021T). Use of this code will help insure that the carriers and the AMA will be able to add it to next year's book.

FOR THE HIGH RISK PATIENT

Finally, if the patient is a high-risk patient and if you are providing services that are above and beyond the normal total obstetrical care services, you will be able to code for these in addition to the code for the total obstetrical care using the appropriate services codes that describe what you did. Make sure that you communicate why you needed these extra services to the insurance company so that you can obtain the appropriate reimbursement.

NERVOUS SYSTEM

As with other subsections of the Surgery Section, the Nervous System is arranged from the top of the head going south. That is, it starts with the skull, meninges and brain and continues with the spine and spinal cord and peripheral nerves.

Many of the codes found in this subsection will require the work of two surgeons working together for the best result for the patient. In these cases, when two physicians both provide parts of one service, each surgeon should use the code number of the service provided and add the modifier –62 for Two Surgeons to the end of the codes. More information about modifiers is found in the chapter on modifiers.

Some of the other nuances of the nervous system include the following:

a. Injection procedures found within this subsection (e.g., 61055, 62273*, 62280, etc.) do not generally include the supply of the material injected. Check with the HCPCS National Codes manual to find the codes for these supplies.

b. There are many codes that are considered "add-on" codes within the nervous system. An example of an add-on code here is the 63035. Make sure that you do not use an add-on code by itself. In other words, make sure that you list the primary service *in addition to* the code for the add-on service. To illustrate this example, suppose a patient had a surgery that included a laminotomy of two interspaces. You would code that in the following way:

63020 *Laminotomy (hemilaminectomy), with decompression of nerve root(s), including partial facetectomy, foraminotomy and/or excision of herniated intervertebral disc; one interspace, cervical*

63035 *each additional interspace, cervical or lumbar (List separately in addition to the code for primary procedure)*

You can see that the first code, 63020, describes the service done on the first interspace. The second or add-on code describes each additional interspace. If you had provided surgeries on more interspaces, you would need to add additional add-on codes as they are appropriate or place the number of additional interspaces in the units column on your claim form. (More information about this will be given when the HCFA 1500 claim form is explained later in this book.)

EYE AND OCULAR ADNEXA

As with many other subsections, the arrangement of this section is from the outer eye inward. Most of the services for the eye listed in the Surgery Section are performed on one eye unless stated otherwise in the description of the code. You will find lots of little notes in and around the codes in this section. Make sure you read them because they will give you clues for more effective coding.

Keep in mind that the codes in this Surgery Section for the eyes only describe invasive services. Diagnostic and noninvasive services provided for the eyes can be found in the Medicine Section of the **CPT** book or can also be found under the Evaluation and Management services, the Radiology Section and the Pathology and Laboratory Section.

Because of the intricate nature of the surgeries performed in this section on the eye, the use of an operating microscope is essential when providing these services. Because an operating microscope is an essential component to providing these services, there is no need to use the code 69990 in addition to the codes found in the Eye and Ocular Adnexa subsections.

Folowing are some of the nuances of the Eye and Ocular Adnexa subsection of Surgery:

a. Similar to laceration repair found in the Integumentary System, repair in the eye itself and its component parts requires that you have the information on both the location of the wound and the type of repair performed. Unlike the Integumentary System, however, the lengths of the repairs are *not* added.

b. Treatment of fractures to the orbital bones are found in the Musculoskeletal System, but incisions and excisions of bone of the orbit are described in the Eye and Ocular Adnexa subsection.

c. If you code for a removal of a foreign body from the eye, even if it is from the conjunctiva (see codes 65205* through 65265), don't forget to code for the x-ray or the echocardiography procedure if you provided these services in order to locate the foreign body.

d. Although you will see codes that are considered to be "separate procedures" in this subsection, it is important to make sure that the codes you choose are in fact separate (distinct) procedures because they are performed on separate (different) parts of the eye and are not components of a larger service. For example, a conjunctival flap, bridge or partial (separate procedure), code 68360, may be part of another service found under the conjunctiva and would not be coded in addition to that other service. Coding for a "separate procedure" is only possible when the "separate procedure" service is not immediately related to the larger more global service. To accomplish this requirement in this case, the "separate procedure" would need used alone or together with a procedure found under a different subsection of the eye (e.g., the Posterior Segment subsection of the Eye and Ocular Adnexa).

e. The supply of an intraocular lens (IOL) is not included with the code for the IOL service itself. If you provide the IOL, you will need to code for it by using one of the HCPCS National Codes.

f. Because of the fact that we are in the surgery section and one eye may require services that another eye does not require, you cannot assume that the codes found in the Eye and Ocular Adnexa subsection are bilateral. In fact, unless otherwise stated within the text of the **CPT** book, you should make the assumption that these codes within the Surgery subsection include services provided to only one eye.

g. Closure of the lacrimal punctum by a plug (68761) is typically done using two plugs. The first service is diagnostic in nature and tests whether or not the closure will even work. It includes a collagen type plug (A4262), the supply of which is not included in with the surgery. If these collagen plugs are effective, permanent plugs (see A4263), are used to replace the collagen ones. This would be a service that is therapeutic in nature. Since the **CPT** code 68761 does not differentiate between the different kinds of plugs and whether or not the service is diagnostic or therapeutic, you may find yourself using the code 68761 twice within a short period of time. Modifier – 76 for Repeat Services may be employed to describe that both operations that ended up being the same **CPT** code were done by the same physician. Another modifier that you may consider using is the modifier – 78 for Return To The Operating Room For A Related Procedure During The Postoperative Period. This could help show that you are well aware of the fact that the procedure is not "duplicate" (e.g., that the first was done as a trail to insure that the second one would work). No codes are needed for the removal of the temporary plugs because they usually dissolve in the puncta. Check with your carrier on its policy regarding the use of the HCPCS codes for supplies. Variations exist on this issue from carrier to carrier.

h. If you see the phrase "one or more sessions" as part of the description of a code, you will need to make sure that the physician has defined the treatment series (the number of times the patient will receive that same service) before you use the code. These words, "one or more sessions," do not mean that you can code the number repeatedly each time you provide the service. An example of this follows:

65855 Trabeculoplasty by laser surgery, one or more sessions (defined treatment series)

Auditory System

There are very few nuances associated with coding for the ear. Among the nuances are the following:

a. Services found in the Auditory System of the Surgery Section are considered to be unilateral unless otherwise stated. That is, unless the code specifically tells you that the service was performed on both ears, you should assume that it was only provided on one. This is due to the fact that we cannot assume just because you need to operate on one ear that you will also need to operate on the other.

b. There are many services within this subsection that are performed using the techniques of an operating microscope. When you use an operating microscope and when it is not already part of the overall service, be sure to employ the code 69990, which indicates that microsurgical techniques were used. You will use this code in addition to the code for the primary surgery(ies), but as per the instructions in the **CPT** book before the code 69990, you will *not* need to add the modifier –51 to the 69990.

c. The removal of tubes from the ear is considered to be part of the postoperative follow-up portion of the surgery. It is not coded separately. If another surgeon placed ventilating tubes and you are the one removing them, use the code 69424, which describes the service of removing ventilating tubes placed by another physician. As stated in the first nuance, unilaterality is assumed in this subsection. If you removed tubes from both ears and did not place those tubes you will need to add the modifier –50 to the second removal in order to show that both ears were treated.

Summary

CHAPTER SEVEN

✓ All codes in the Surgery Section begin with a 1, 2, 3, 4, 5, or 6.

✓ It is important that you read and understand the Surgery guidelines.

✓ According to **CPT**, non-starred surgical procedures (Surgical Package) include the following:

- Local infiltration, metacarpal/metatarsal, digital block or topical anesthesia when used;
- One related E/M code immediately prior to or on the date of surgery. (This does not include the E/M visit during which the decision to operate was made.);
- The operation per se;
- Normal, uncomplicated follow-up care.

✓ For many carriers, the "carrier" Surgical Package includes the following:

- Pre-op
- Surgery
- Post-op

✓ For Medicare, the Surgical Package concept (known as the National Global Surgery Policy) includes the following:

- Visits no more than one day prior to surgery, not including the one during which it was decided that the patient would receive surgery;
- Surgery;
- Complications that do not require a trip back to the operating room;
- Post-op care from zero through ninety days.

✓ For Medicare, the visit at which the decision to operate was made is a billable service. Addition of the modifier -57 to the end of the E/M code (pre-op) may be helpful.

✓ Another modifier you may consider using to indicate an E/M service that occurred prior to a "surgery" (especially in the case of minor surgical procedures like starred services) would be the modifier –25 for Significant, Separately Identifiable E/M Service By The Same Physician on the Same Day of the Procedure or Other Service.

- ✓ The price for non-starred surgical procedures should reflect all components of the Surgical Package (i.e., each of the three components).

- ✓ According to **CPT**, any complications or exacerbations of the surgery are not included in the Surgical Package, and procedures performed to correct or alleviate these problems should be coded separately.

- ✓ According to Medicare, complications that do not require a revisit to the operating room are included in with the price of the surgery.

- ✓ Because normal, uncomplicated follow-up care is included with the total surgical package in **CPT**, you should use the 99024 code with no charge to indicate the patient's follow-up visits.

- ✓ It is important to know the number of follow-up days that your carrier includes with each Surgical Package and to bill for the Office/Outpatient or Hospital visits made thereafter. Many carriers have a set number of follow-up days that are the same for all non-starred surgical services, and this number is important to know. Check with your carrier.

✓ The number of follow-up days for surgeries done to Medicare patients ranges from 0 - 90 days, depending on the surgery. A list of these days and the corresponding **CPT** code numbers has been published by Medicare.

✓ According to **CPT**, follow-up care for diagnostic services includes only care that relates to the diagnostic procedure itself; it does not include care for the condition for which the procedure was initially performed.

✓ According to **CPT** rules, the physician who provides supplies may choose to bill for supplies and materials over and above those usually included with the office/outpatient visit or other services rendered.

✓ According to Medicare rules, supplies and materials above and beyond those usually included with the service may be listed in addition to the codes if they fall within the services that Medicare outlined for these additional supplies.

✓ It is important to list multiple procedures occurring on the same day with separate entries, as long as they are not part of the overall global service (i.e., as long as they do not have the words "separate procedure" following the description in **CPT**).

✓ Multiple procedures should be placed on the claim form in order **from major to minor service**, with a separate price listed for each service.

✓ The words "*separate procedure*" mean that you can bill for it only when that procedure is performed alone (not as part of the larger or more global service) or for a specific purpose. More information on separate procedures can be found in the Surgery Section in the guidelines of **CPT**.

✓ It is important to read all of the notes in any subsection as well as any paragraph written for which you cannot find an existing procedure code.

✓ When using an "unlisted procedure" code, make sure that you submit a special report explaining to the claims processor in layman's terms the unusual circumstances of the service.

✓ In coding a starred procedure, remember that you are coding only for the surgical service itself and that you should strive to complete the Surgical Package by coding separately for any pre-op, regional or general anesthesia, and post-op components provided.

✓ The Surgery Section is arranged (for the most part) from outside the body (Integumentary System) inward (Musculoskeletal, Respiratory, Cardiovascular Systems, etc.).

✓ Three different kinds of repairs are listed in the Integumentary System section/subsection.

1. Simple repair .... Single layer closure
2. Intermediate repair .... Layer closure
3. Complex repair .... Plastic/cosmetic repair

✓ When coding repairs in the Integumentary System, you should measure and record the size of the lesion in centimeters including conservative margins and measured using the diameter at the widest portion of the lesion before it is excised, and code the repair according to its type (simple, intermediate, or complex).

✓ Repairs in the Integumentary System of the same classification and location (as given in the description of the code) should be added together and reported as a single item.

✓ In coding for the first fracture repair where *treatment* of the fracture is involved, make sure to use the codes found between 20000* and 28899.

✓ Codes found between 29000 and 29799 are used for second- or third-time placement of a cast or for first-time cast placement done for the purpose of stabilizing or protecting the bone.

✓ Re-reduction of a fracture by the same physician should be indicated by placing a -76 modifier following the procedure code number. Re-reduction by a different physician should be indicated by placing a -77 following the procedure code number.

✓ Codes found to cover total obstetrical care include all care on a prenatal, birth and postnatal basis that are normal and uncomplicated.

✓ Complications during pregnancy, such as toxemia or preterm labor, can be coded in addition to the codes for the total obstetrical care, using the appropriate codes to describe the services.

✓ The services for codes found in the Nervous System are commonly provided by two physicians. Each physician should report the service(s) he or she provides, and if the services are performed jointly and with each physician maintaining a 50% role in the surgery using the same **CPT** code, both physicians can report the procedure with the addition of the modifier –62 (Two Surgeons) on the end of the Surgery code.

- ✓ Codes found in the Auditory and Eye and Ocular Adnexa systems of the Surgery Section are considered to be one-sided (unilateral) unless stated otherwise in the description of the code. To show that the codes were done bilaterally, you would need to add the modifier –50 for Bilateral services to the end of the code.

- ✓ Microsurgery is an inherent part of the codes found in the Eye and Ocular Adnexa subsection. Use of a modifier to describe the microsurgery or use of a separate **CPT** code to describe the microsurgery is not warranted.

- ✓ Microsurgery is not an inherent part of the codes found in the Auditory System in Surgery Section. If you provided services using an operating microscope and if the code does not indicate that the services included an operating microscope, you will need to use the code 69990.

- ✓ Codes that apply to the removal of adenoids and tonsils are considered to be bilateral. There is no need to code the number using the modifier –50 for Bilateral services.

- ✓ Codes dealing with bronchoscopy include the inspection of both lungs.

CHAPTER EIGHT

RADIOLOGY

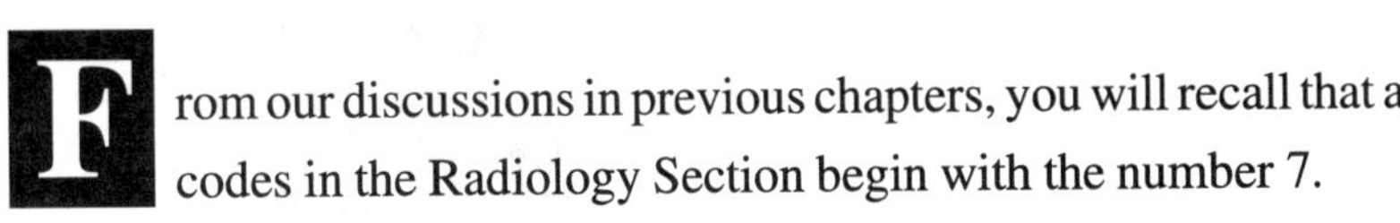

From our discussions in previous chapters, you will recall that all codes in the Radiology Section begin with the number 7.

The Radiology Section is divided into four basic subsections:

- Diagnostic Radiology/Diagnostic Imaging
- Diagnostic Ultrasound
- Radiation Oncology
- Nuclear Medicine

You can tell that these are the four major subsections of the Radiology Section when you look through the **CPT** book and see that it is these four subsections that are highlighted in black headings within the **CPT** text.

These subsections are arranged, for the most part, in alphabetical order. That is, **D**iagnostic Radiology/Diagnostic Imaging is followed by **D**iagnostic Ultrasound, which is followed by **R**adiation Oncology. The Radiology Section ends with Nuclear Medicine (the only subsection that is **not** in alphabetical order).

Within each subsection, codes are arranged, for the most part, in anatomical order, from the top of the body to the bottom (i.e., head and neck, chest, spine, and pelvis).

In Radiology the codes in the subsections have been arranged in anatomical order from top to bottom, i.e., head and neck, chest, spine and pelvis.

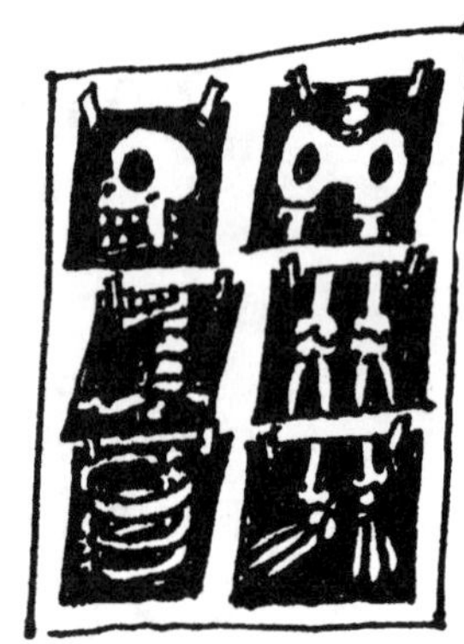

General Rules For Coding Services In Radiology

If you know what kind of procedure your physician performed and if it was performed for diagnostic purposes (to determine the patient's problem) or as part of the patient's treatment, you will be able to find the appropriate subsection. For example, if the x-rays were taken because it was thought that the patient might have a broken arm, you would look in the Diagnostic Radiology subsection because you want to "diagnose" the problem. If, on the other hand, you were trying to eradicate a tumor, you would go to the Radiation Oncology subsection where "treatment" of these conditions can be found. If you know the body part on which the procedure was performed, you will be able to find the appropriate code within that subsection.

The Radiology Section begins with guidelines like all other sections in **CPT** and concludes with a complete listing of all procedure codes applicable to radiology.

As is true of services discussed in other sections of **CPT**, you can appropriately code for multiple radiologic services rendered on the same day with separate listings.

If a service your physician is providing cannot be found among the listings in **CPT**, you can use one of the unlisted service or procedure codes found at the end of each subsection and also in the unlisted service or procedure guidelines at the beginning of the Radiology Section.

If you find it necessary to use an unlisted procedure code, it is important that you remember to submit a special report with your claim so that the claims processor will be able to understand the procedure(s) provided and reimburse your office accordingly.

In submitting a special report, keep in mind that you are communicating with someone who may have had very little exposure to medical terminology. The less complicated your report is written (i.e., the more in "layman's terms" it is written), the better your chances for optimal reimbursement.

CPT suggests that your special report include the following:

Special Report
• Complexity of symptoms • Final diagnosis • Pertinent physical findings • Diagnostic and therapeutic procedures • Concurrent problems • Follow-up care

Finally, if you want to code for something for which there is no existing code, you may consider using the unlisted procedure code, 79999, or finding a code from the Category III codes (if there is one) or one that comes close to describing the procedure or service your physician provided (although it may not be exact), adding modifier -22 (the Unusual Service modifier) and submitting a special report with your claim. If you choose this method, the data entry person at the carrier's office will pass the claim along to a supervisor for manual review, possibly delaying your payment.

hint

Another suggestion: Rather than using an unlisted procedure code, check with your carrier to see if another code has been invented to describe the procedure. You may also want to check the ***National Coding Manual (HCPCS Level II)*** *if the patient is a Medicare patient or try locating the code in the Category III section of codes.*

COMPLETE PROCEDURES

The Radiology Section contains listings that contain the terminology "complete procedure". These are radiologic services that include all views of a certain area.

Here is an example of a complete procedure:

> *72114 Radiologic examination, spine, lumbosacral; complete, including bending views*

Notice that all views of the spine and lumbosacral areas are included with this procedure code.

SUPERVISION AND INTERPRETATION

The 1991 and prior versions of **CPT** featured the phrase "complete procedure" to include (a) the procedures themselves (e.g., endoscopy or injection of a contrast medium) and (b) supervision and interpretation of those procedures. This definition is no longer used.

Effective with the 1992 version of **CPT**, codes in the Radiology Section (with the exception of those in the Radiation Oncology subsection) describe only the supervision and interpretation of procedures and do NOT include such things as the injection of the contrast media or the placement of the scope for endoscopy. Supervision implies that the physician is available during the procedure for any assistance that the technician may need. Interpretation is the reading of the results of the films. The procedures themselves (e.g., endoscopy or injection of a contrast medium) are coded in other sections of the book (usually the Surgery Section). Therefore, the meaning of "complete procedures," as it related to supervision, interpretation, and injection or endoscopy from previous versions of **CPT,** would not apply. The following is an example of a code for supervision and interpretation:

75820 Venography, extremity, unilateral radiological supervision and interpretation

If one physician performed the procedure (see 36000, 36005, 36406, 36410, 36420, 36425 for the surgical portion of the complete procedure) and another provided supervision and interpretation, each would code the service he or she provided. If the same physician provided both services (the procedure itself, plus supervision and interpretation), he or she would use two codes, one for the procedure (usually found in the Surgery Section) and the other for supervision and interpretation (Radiology Section).

As with any other sections of **CPT**, new codes in Radiology are denoted with a bullet (●) and revised descriptions are preceded with a triangle (▲). Any new or revised "non-descriptive" text is indicated using the inverted triangles (▸ ◂). Radiology uses add-on codes (✚) which indicate additional procedures done at the same time by the same physician and which are part of the primary procedure performed.

As with other sections of **CPT**, reading the "notes" surrounding those codes is always important. The notes will give you insight into the proper and accurate coding of procedures and services in the Radiology Section.

Let's look at some examples of how to code with the Radiology Section. Let's say that your physician is an orthopedic surgeon who has an x-ray machine on the premises. A patient comes into your office (at the request of the local pediatrician) for you to render an opinion on the status of the patient's back (e.g., for you to tell the pediatrician whether or not the patient has scoliosis). Your office technician takes the x-rays, develops them and gives the film to your doctor, who reads the films and diagnoses scoliosis for the patient. You would first ask yourself, into which of the following basic groups does the service our office provided fall?

a. Diagnostic Radiology
b. Diagnostic Ultrasound
c. Therapeutic Radiology
d. Nuclear Medicine

It is easy to see that the service you provided was of the first category and that it was clearly diagnostic in nature (i.e., you wanted to find out what was wrong, if anything, with the patient). In making the decision where to look for the kind of service you performed, you can see that it would be located in the Diagnostic Radiology subsection of the Radiology Section. As you will recall from the discussion at the beginning of this chapter, much of the Radiology Section is arranged from top to bottom within a particular subsection. In other words, the Diagnostic Radiology subsection is arranged starting with **H**ead and **N**eck and continuing down the body. Since the service we provided was located on the back, you would look towards the middle of the Diagnostic Radiology subsection under Spine and Pelvis. As you can see (if you are following along with me in your **CPT** book), the probable code would be the following:

> *72069 Radiologic examination, spine, thoracolumbar, standing (scoliosis)*

Additionally, you should consider code 72090 which also describes scoliosis. The difficulty with this example is that you don't have enough information here to know which code more closely resembles the service you provided. Remember, if you provided a consultation where you evaluated the patient in an office-like setting, you need to code the number for that service (see E/M codes) in addition to the code for the x-ray.

Take another example. Let's say that the same patient came into your office for your opinion on whether or not she had scoliosis, but this time, she brought films done by another physician. You could still review these films, but you would not charge any "extra" for the review because the service of reviewing past medical data is considered part of the Evaluation and Management service, under the decision-making component. (You may recall that there are three key components to most Evaluation and Management services. These include the history, exam and medical decision-making. Medical decision-making requires you to consider the number of diagnosis or management options, the risk of mobility or mortality and the amount and/or complexity of data to be reviewed. The review of these films, taken by someone else, falls into the category of Amount and/or Complexity of Data to be Reviewed.) The only code you could use, therefore, for the patient who presents herself with her past data or films is to code for the service(s) you provide. Since in this case, you only provided the consultation (see E/M Consultation codes), that is the service for which you would code and bill.

Another form of "consultation" exists in **CPT** Radiology Section. This is the code 76140.

76140 *Consultation on x-ray examination made elsewhere, written report*

This code, 76140, is used when the radiologist receives a film from another doctor and when the radiologist is asked to render his opinion and prepare a written report. Notice that the description does not say anything about the patient being present, so you cannot assume that the patient is present. If the patient were present, you would use the consultation codes from the Evaluation and Management Section. Another note of importance here is the portion of the description that describes a written report. If your physician reviews a film and does not prepare a written report, she cannot use this consultation code, 76140, but would need to use the **CPT** code describing the x-ray examination with a modifier–26 for Professional Component. The addition of this modifier to the **CPT** code would let the carrier know that a reading was provided on the film.

In another scenario, suppose a boy comes to the hospital following a fight that occurred at a local school. The boy is admitted to the emergency room and is complaining of a bloody and painful nose. The hospital x-rays the patient and completes a 3-view x-ray of both the nasal bones. The radiologist reports a diagnosis of displacement of the nasal septum.

In coding for this example, you would need to make sure what position you were in (as the coder). For example, if you were employed by the physician, you would need to report the code for the x-ray of the nasal bones with a modifier to indicate that your physician "read" the films even though she did not provide the "technical component" (e.g., your physician did not "take" the x-rays).

Consider another example. Let us say that you work for an OB/GYN. A patient comes into your office and presents herself for her annual physical. Upon examination, you notice that there appears to be a mass in the lower left side of her abdomen. You palpate some more and decide that it would be best to get an ultrasound of the area to see what is going on. Your technician takes the patient down the hall and completes an ultrasound of the lower left quadrant. You code the service with the following code:

76705 *Ultrasound, abdominal, B-scan and/or real time with image documentation; limited (e.g., single organ, quadrant, follow-up)*

In the above case, you are the one providing the technical and professional component and can code the service as it is listed above.

When you are performing angiographies, the story is somewhat different. As you can see by looking at the codes for Aorta and Arteries (look before the code subsection starting with the number 75600), most of the codes in this subsection of Radiology include only the supervision and interpretation of the procedure. However, there are instances where your physician will perform the intravenous or intraarterial procedure. In these cases, the **CPT** book refers you to the Surgery Section to pick up the "invasive" portion of the service.

To illustrate this, say your patient needs to get a thoracic aortography (without serialography). Let's also suppose that your radiologist performs both the supervision and interpretation of the service as well as the procedure for injection of the catheter into the superior vena cava. You would code for both services using the following:

36010 *Introduction of catheter, superior or inferior vena cava*

75600 *Aortography, thoracic, without serialography, radiologic supervision and interpretation*

Notice that you use both codes to completely delineate the service.

MAMMOGRAPHY

When you find yourself needing to use the codes for breast studies (see codes 76086 through 76096), keep in mind that you must be careful to use the code that describes the sides for which you provided the mammogram. For example, if you only did a mammogram on one side, you would use the code for "unilateral" mammogram. If you provided mammograms on both breasts, you would choose the code that describes the bilateral procedure. Under no circumstances would you use the modifier –50 for Bilateral services when you already have a specific code that describes the service(s).

Although there are many codes that describe procedures to the breast, most of them are straightforward. The main thing to keep in mind with the breasts is the different forms of testing that may be done. For example you may see a code that describes a "*screening*" mammogram. The word "*screening*" implies that the patient has not reported any problems and that the test is done either to get a baseline or to make sure that the patient is free of any disease. You may also see "*screening*" applying to images of each breast in two projections from the head down (craniocaudal), and from side to side (mediolateral). If you do not see the word "*screening*", you will know that the code includes the diagnosis of some sort of condition.

Diagnostic Ultrasound

The terminology in this subsection is often confusing to first-time coders and those not familiar with radiology services. Let us take a brief review of some of the terminology in order to gain a better understanding of this subsection.

- **A-mode:** A one-dimensional picture with no movement of the device (trace) held by the technician or radiologist. An example would be a view of the breast where no tissues or structures are moving.

- **M-mode:** A one-dimensional view of a structure (or structures) where the trace is moving across the structure(s) in an effort to get the scope of the structure (amplitude) as well as the quickness of motion (velocity) if the structure is moving. An example of this might be the view of a fetus that is moving within the mother.

- **B-scan:** A two-dimensional scan with a two-dimensional display.

- **Real-time scan:** Similar to the M-mode scan, in which you obtain the amplitude of the structure and the velocity (motion), only in this case you obtain a two-dimensional view of the specimen(s) with time.

Once you have decided which kind of ultrasound was provided, you can select the appropriate **CPT** code with little or no problems. Remember, like many other subsections in **CPT**, you will find the arrangement of this one going from the head to the toes.

RADIATION ONCOLOGY

Radiation Oncology is one of the broadest sections of the Radiology Chapter because of the intensity of the services and the uniqueness of the treatment based on the needs of the different patients. It is not the scope of this book to detail each and every component of this subsection that you will need to know. However, a background in understanding the generalities of the subsection will go a long way towards helping you code these services if you find yourself employed by a radiologist or hospital.

In general, the codes listed here are divided into various subsections. The first of these includes the consultation or clinical management of the patient. Keep in mind that when a patient initially comes to see a radiation oncologist, the visit could very well be coded using the codes from the Evaluation and Management Section. Think of this like you think of a surgeon trying to decide whether or not she should operate on a patient. If you think about what is involved, you will agree that the surgeon must assess the patient, get a history, find out the current issues and make a plan according to the specific needs of the patient. The same is true here. The radiation oncologist will assess the patient by obtaining a full history, performing an exam, and reviewing past lab results and/or results of other tests (including x-rays and ultrasounds), and make a decision on how to proceed. All of these services can and should be coded with the Evaluation and Management codes (see 99201 - 99275). Once a decision has been made that the patient does in fact require the services of the radiation oncologist, the physician will proceed in preparing a plan of action for the treatment of the patient. When this happens, you can use the codes found in the **CPT** book, in the Radiology Section (see codes 77261-77263). These are the codes that will describe various levels of difficulty in the planning process (e.g., where to place the radiation treatment portals, how long the treatment should be).

Once treatment begins and is delivered, you will notice that the treatment is delivered in amounts or MeV's. MeV's are the measurement units of the amount of energy used to treat the patient. Make sure that you understand and can report the number of MeV's before deciding upon a code.

When you begin to use the codes found under the Radiation Treatment Management subsection you will need to be aware of the fact that these codes use the term "*fractions*" to signify the number of treatment sessions. Although this may sound bothersome at first, keep in mind that patients may receive multiple treatments in a day or during a week. Knowing that the basic "*fraction*" is equal to five treatments can help you in your coding. The amount of time spent during a particular treatment session does not matter. The only thing counted is the session itself, regardless of the amount of time spent during the session.

Let's take an example. Suppose you treated a patient using two treatment sessions on Monday and then another two sessions three days later, on Thursday. (The total number of sessions does not yet make up one fraction because you need five treatments to make up one fraction.) When the patient came back on the following Monday and you delivered another session, you would be able to code the following:

77427 Radiation treatment management, five treatments

Try to come as close as you can to the five treatment sessions before using any of these treatment codes. Carriers, as well as the AMA, frown upon using the code above if you only provided one treatment (or 1/5 of a fraction).

You will also see services listed for Proton Beam therapy (using beams of protons as opposed to regular forms of radiation to treat the area), Hyperthermia (using heat to raise the temperature of a specific area in an attempt to increase the cell metabolism and thereby kill the tumor), and Clinical Bradytherapy (where the radioactive sources are placed directly into the tumor-bearing area to generate well–defined regions of high intensity radiation to kill the tumor). The codes here are fairly self-explanatory and should be carefully read before employing a code.

NUCLEAR MEDICINE

Nuclear medicine involves the placement of radionuclides within the body (e.g., the thyroid or heart) and then watching how these radionuclides emit their waste (radioactive elements) within the different tissues. By the way that an organ or tumor accepts or rejects the waste, physicians can tell what is wrong with the patient or they can determine the extent of the tumor. For example, they can determine whether areas are diseased or healthy by the amount of radionuclides accepted by the tissues. Doctors can also use nuclear medicine techniques to treat patients.

Selection of a code (or codes) within this subsection is simple as the selection is based upon what system you are providing services for (e.g., if you are providing services to the Endocrine System go look there, the same is true for the Hematopoietic, Reticuloendothelial and Lymphatic Systems). You will need to locate the system first and then find the code or codes that best suit your situation. Note that at the end of the Nuclear Medicine subsection is a place where you can find codes for "therapeutic" type Nuclear Radiology services. These codes are separate from the other Nuclear Medicine codes that are more diagnostic in nature.

Use of Modifier -50, Bilateral Services in Radiology

Although the modifier –50 Bilateral services (see the Chapter on Modifiers to learn more), there may or may not be a need to employ it in the Radiology Section. It bears repeating to say that many of the code descriptions in the Radiology Section already use the term bilateral and have assigned a specific code number to the description for bilateral services. Not only that, many carriers, including Medicare, prefer that you use other modifiers than the –50 to indicate the fact that your service applied to both sides of the body. (As you already know from the discussion on HCPCS National Codes, there are alpha-modifiers (modifiers that are all letters and not numbers like in **CPT**), that are used by many insurance carriers. Modifiers to keep in mind when you are coding for equal services that are performed on both sides of the body are the –RT, for services performed on the right side and the –LT, for service performed on the left side).

Summary

CHAPTER EIGHT

✓ Codes in the Radiology Section begin with the number 7.

✓ The four subsections in the Radiology Section include:

- Diagnostic Radiology
- Diagnostic Ultrasound
- Radiation Oncology
- Nuclear Medicine

✓ The codes in the subsections are generally arranged by anatomic site, from the top of the body to the bottom.

✓ Complete procedures are those that include all views of a certain area.

✓ If a physician provides supervision and interpretation of a procedure, as well as performs the procedure itself (e.g., endoscopy, injection of a contrast medium), two codes should be used, one for the procedure itself and the other for supervision and interpretation of the procedure.

✓ Codes for the procedures such as injection of contrast media for endoscopy are found in other sections of **CPT**, usually the Surgery Section. Codes for supervision and interpretation of the procedures are found in the Radiology Section.

✓ It is important to read all of the notes in each subsection, as they give important information about accurate coding of the procedures found in that subsection.

✓ Check with your carrier before using the modifier –50 for Bilateral services on the end of a procedure code. You should also check all of the codes to make sure that one of them doesn't already describe a bilateral service.

✓ Radiation treatment management is measured in "fractions," where a fraction is equal to five treatments.

✓ There are consultations found in the Radiology Section. These include looking at x-rays that were prepared elsewhere, forming an opinion about the films and preparing a written report.

CHAPTER NINE

PATHOLOGY AND LABORATORY

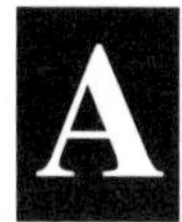
ll codes in the Pathology and Laboratory Section of **CPT** begin with the number 8.

Coding for the services in the Pathology Section is similar to coding for services found elsewhere in the **CPT** book. That is, you determine which services were provided, decide what kind of services were done (e.g., services on blood, urine, chemistry-type services) and then locate the code(s).

This section, like all others in **CPT**, begins with guidelines and then lists procedures and services applicable to the field of pathology.

Services listed in the Pathology and Laboratory Section are those provided either by a technician under a physician's supervision or by the physician (usually a pathologist). As with other sections of the book, it is appropriate to list as many multiple services as were rendered to the patient on the same day, given that they are not otherwise combined under a larger, more global service (for example, Organ or Disease-Oriented Panels) which group several tests together under one code.

hint

It is very important that you understand the information contained in the notes before you begin to code the procedures and services found in each subsection.

INSTRUCTIONS

You will find that there are many notes that come in and around the codes in the Pathology Section. These usually include some sort of special instructions that need to be considered when coding the numbers in and around the subsection in which they appear. It is vital that you understand the information contained here before you begin to code procedures and services found in these subsections.

The following subsections make a special point of listing notes:

- Organ or Disease-Oriented Panels
- Drug Testing
- Therapeutic Drug Assays
- Evocative/Suppression Testing
- Consultations

- Urinalysis
- Chemistry
- Hematology and Coagulation
- Immunology
- Transfusion Medicine
- Microbiology
- Anatomic Pathology
- Cytopathology
- Cytogenic Studies
- Surgical Pathology
- Transcutaneous Procedures
- Other Procedures

UNLISTED PROCEDURES

As in other sections of **CPT**, unlisted procedures are found in the Pathology and Laboratory Section. If you are unable to find a procedure you wish to describe, follow these steps:

1. Look in the **HCPCS National Coding Manual** (Level II) for the code(s) if the patient is a Medicare, Medicaid or SCHIP patient and if the carrier to which the claim will be submitted can accept Level II codes.

or

2. Use an unlisted procedure code in the appropriate subsection (e.g., Urinalysis, Chemistry and Toxicology, and

Hematology) or, if at all possible, find an appropriate code in the Category III section of the **CPT** book, which is located right before the appendices, towards the back of the **CPT** manual. If you are using an unlisted procedure, be sure to submit a special report with your claim *so that the carrier will know what you are trying to code.*

or

3. *Ask for assignment of a special number* by that carrier to fit the procedure or service you wish to describe.

or

4. Choose a procedure that comes close to the procedure for which you would like to bill and add modifier -22 (Unusual Service modifier).

Special Reports

When you use modifier -22, the data entry person at the carrier's office will not be able to process your claim; he or she will have to refer it to a claims supervisor for review. Modifier -22 indicates that the service provided is different from anything found in the latest version of **CPT**. In most (but not all) cases, the person who submitted the claim is requesting additional payment because of unusual circumstances surrounding the service provided.

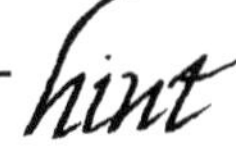

When submitting a claim with modifier -22, you must also submit a special report. In submitting this report, you need to explain the procedure in simple terms so that the person processing your claim will understand what you are trying to code.

In submitting a special report, it is important not only that you make the report understandable to the claims processor, but **CPT** suggests that you also include the following:

SPECIAL REPORT
• Complexity of symptoms • Final diagnosis • Pertinent physical findings • Diagnostic and therapeutic procedures • Concurrent problems • Follow-up care

SUBSECTION ARRANGEMENTS

Within each subsection of the Pathology Section, the descriptions of the codes are, for the most part, arranged alphabetically. For example, in checking the subsection on Chemistry, you will see that it begins with codes describing tests for acetaldehyde (82000), acetaminophen (82003), and so on.

It is important for you to browse through and become familiar with the last subsections of the Pathology and Laboratory Section. Read the descriptions of procedures found in the subsections on Anatomic and Surgical Pathology, as well as those found in the miscellaneous codes subsection. These contain codes such as gastric and nasal smears and semen analysis, to name a few.

When you are coding using the Pathology and Laboratory Section, remember that the collection of the specimen is not included as part of the codes found here. That is, the 80000 series of codes does not include the obtaining of the specimen that is tested unless otherwise stated in the notes surrounding that subsection or within the description of the code. The 80000 series of codes includes the test itself. In general, you can assume that if the specimen was in liquid format (e.g., blood, urine, cerebrospinal fluid), the description of the code will not include the collection of such a specimen and you will need to look to another section of the **CPT** book (often the Surgery Section) to get a code for the collection (if you provided the service of collection). If you are providing the pathology and laboratory test as well as obtaining the specimen, you will need to code for both.

There is still a debate over which code to use for Medicare patients who reccive blood draws (commonly known in **CPT** as "routinc venipuncture"). The AMA suggests use of the code 36415* to report the venipuncture. Medicare, probably due to the fact that the 36415* is a starred surgical service and would therefore qualify to be coded as such (see rules for coding starred services in the Surgery Section), asks that the coder employ the code G0001 for the routine venipuncture for collection of specimen. Be sure to look at the kind of insurance your patient has before selecting the 36514* or the G0001.

Three subsections of the Pathology and Laboratory Section have some unusual nuances of which you need to be aware. These nuances are found in the following subsections:

- Organ or Disease-Oriented Panels
- Drug Testing
- Surgical Pathology

We will take each of these subsections and explore the special nuances within each of them.

Organ or Disease-Oriented Panels

Each of the the Organ or Disease-Oriented Panels was defined to include certain tests. For example, a general health panel (i.e., 80050) includes the following:

80050 *General health panel*

1. Comprehensive metabolic panel (80053);

plus

2. a. Hemogram, automated and manual differential WBC count (CBC) (85022);

or

b. Hemogram and platelet count, automated and automated complete differential WBC count (CBC) (85025);

and

3. Thyroid stimulating hormone (TSH) (84443).

In order to report a code for a particular panel, all of the tests as outlined in the description of the code must be performed. No cafeteria style is available here; you can't just go through and pick out what you want from the description and leave the rest.

An extensive rewrite of the Organ and Disease-Oriented Panels was made available with the 1998 **CPT** book. Note that each of the panels found in the Organ or Disease-Oriented Panel subsection includes combinations of tests that can occur separately or together with one another. When coding using these "panel" codes, pay special attention to the words "or" and "and" as they will tell you what is *or is not* included in the test.

If you are performing other tests in addition to those listed in the panel, you need to report them separately. If you do not perform the tests required and defined as part of this code, you cannot use the code and will need to look elsewhere for a number that more accurately describes your service.

Drug Testing

Drugs such as alcohol, amphetamines, barbiturates, and many others can be detected in two ways:

a. Quantitatively
b. Qualitatively

Quantitative detection tells the pathologist *how much* of the drug is present in the person's body.

Qualitative detection tells the physician *if* a drug is present in the person's body (i.e., which drugs can be found in the patient?).

You may find yourself using both quantitative and qualitative tests. For example, you may discover that a person has a certain drug in her body and then you may need to know how much of the drug she has in her body.

Pay attention to words like "each procedure" as you may find yourself having to use the same code number more than once.

For example:

80100 *Drug screen, qualitative; multiple drug classes chromatographic method, each procedure*

You will need to use this code *each time* you test for another drug class.

The Drug Testing subsection in the Pathology Section of **CPT** aims at giving codes for the qualitative detection of drugs. The pathology lab uses tests such as chromatography to confirm that the drug was present.

If the physician needs to know how much of a drug (or drugs) is present in the patient, the lab will need to use the codes under the Chemistry or Therapeutic Drug Assay subsection.

Evocative/Suppression Testing

The codes found within this section range from 80400 through 80440. The tests found here are used to measure how different body parts are working (e.g., whether or not the pituitary gland is working properly). To do this, the pathologist will either administer different agents to "evoke" (or call forth) certain things (analytes) (e.g., ACTH, Calcitonin) or suppress (restrain) them (e.g., Aldosterone, Dexamethasone). Since, as was discussed before, the codes in the 80000 series include only the tests themselves, it will be important to keep in mind that if your physician administered the evocative or suppressive agents, he or she will need to code separately for the administration of these agents and for the supply of the agent(s) (see HCPCS National Codes for the supply of these agents and codes 90780-90784 for the administration of these agents).

For example, if a physician wanted to test the body for adrenal insufficiency, and he infused a substance to test for that, he may order an ACTH stimulation panel. The codes for this test, drug and infusion would be the following:

80400	*ACTH stimulation panel; for adrenal insufficiency*
	This panel must include the following:
	Cortisol (82533 x 2)
90780	*Intravenous infusion for therapy/diagnosis, administered by physician or under direct supervision of physician; up to one hour*
J____	*Supply of analytic agent*

As you can see by reading the description listed above, the test requires that you test for this analyte (substance) two times (that is why you will use 80400, which includes both tests). In using this code 80400, you would not use the code 82533 two times because using the code 80400 is the same as using the code 82533 twice. This test requires two measures because the level of substance being tested for may vary in the blood at different times. By obtaining multiple specimens, even minutes apart, and then combining these and taking the test twice (in this case), you can obtain a better baseline for what the true results really are.

Pathology Consultations

If you were to examine the Pathology and Laboratory Section completely, you would notice that there are three areas where the **CPT** book lists consultations. These include the following:

a. Consultations found under Clinical Pathology (see codes 80500-80502);

b. Consultations on referred material (see codes 88321-88325);

c. Consultations during surgery (see codes 88329-88332).

Consultations under Clinical Pathology

Let's say that a patient has come to your office with a history of a lot of physical and chemical problems, among them, thyroid problems, cancer and diabetes. The tests ordered all measure for the items that need to be measured, but when the results are returned to the physician, it is noted that many of the tests come back borderline and it is impossible to say whether or not the drugs given to the patient are doing their job. The attending physician decides to send these results (obtained from a few labs) to the pathologist at the main hospital and ask for her opinion about the effectiveness of the treatment based on the patient's condition.

The pathologist reviews the patient's past medical history via a copy of the patient's complete chart and reviews the lab results as well. This pathologist would code the following:

80502 *Clinical pathology consultation; comprehensive, for a complex diagnostic problem, with review of patient's history and medical records*

Consultations on Referred Material

Let's take an example of another kind of consultation. Suppose a patient went to see a family practitioner in a small town for a skin rash that had not cleared up for some time. Let's also say that this patient is 75 years old and that this rash started about 2 months ago and has not cleared up and does not seem to be responding to any treatment. The physician decides to take a specimen of the patient's skin and send it to the pathologist to determine what may be the cause of the problem. When the specimen is sent over to the lab, the pathologist prepares slides from the specimen given, analyzes them and prepares a report for the attending physician.

The pathologist could employ the code 88323 from the Consultations on Referred Material subsection (see 88321-88325) to code and bill for the services he performed.

88323 *Consultation and report on referred material requiring preparation of slides*

You could also use these codes for a consultation that was provided on materials from another lab or even in the same facility.

Surgical Pathology

The last kind of consultation to discuss here is the kind of consultation that occurs during surgery. For example:

88300 LEVEL I - Surgical pathology, gross examination only

To correctly read the above code, you need to understand the term "gross." According to Dorland's Medical Dictionary, gross means:

Gross: *"coarse or large; visible to the naked eye, as gross pathology; macroscopic; taking no account minutiae."*

Gross examination would cover that which is visible to the naked eye. Code 88300 describes any specimen that can be examined without the use of a microscope. Compare the 88300 code to the next one.

88302 LEVEL II - Surgical pathology, gross and microscopic examination

- *Appendix, Incidental*
- *Fallopian Tube, Sterilization*
- *Fingers/Toes, Amputation, Traumatic*
- *Foreskin, Newborn*
- *Hernia Sac, Any Location*
- *Hydrocele Sac*
- *Nerve*
- *Skin, Plastic Repair*
- *Sympathetic Ganglion*
- *Testis, Castration*
- *Vaginal Mucosa, Incidental*
- *Vas Deferens, Sterilization*

As you can see by the description of this code, the pathologist uses both the regular (gross) examination and the microscopic one to completely examine the specimen. The code also limits the kind of specimen that may be seen at this particular level. For example, if you performed a gross and microscopic examination on an appendix for a patient who had surgery due to an acute appendicitis, you could not code the 88302 because this code includes the gross and microscopic exam of an appendix that was taken incidentally. You would need to use the code 88304, which includes the exam for an appendix being studied for reasons other than incidental ones. Note that the degree of pathology is greater as we move up the levels in the Surgical Pathology subsection.

Notice that each code from 88300 through 88309 is a "*level.*" Each *level* represents the degree of difficulty involved in the physician's evaluation of a particular specimen, as well as the type of tissue being examined and whether the test was done under gross and microscopic examination. Before coding the evaluation of any specimen, it is important that you read and understand what kind of specimen was evaluated and whether it was inspected by both gross and microscopic examination as opposed to microscopic examination only or gross examination only. Knowing this information will help you select the correct code.

Last but not least, let's take one more example. Pretend you are a surgeon who is operating on a person who has breast tumors. During the surgery, you open the patient and remove what you think are the tumors. While the patient remains under anesthesia, these are sent up to the lab to make sure that you have obtained clear margins (that you got the entire tumor out). The pathologist who reviews your specimen(s) would code in the following way:

88307 Level IV- Surgical pathology, gross and microscopic examination breast excision of lesion, requiring microscopic evaluation of surgical margins

Urinalysis

Now that we have finished talking about the kinds of consultations available within the Pathology Section, let's move back to following the order of the codes as per their arrangement in the **CPT** book.

The codes found in the Urinalysis subsection range from 81000 through 81099. Most of the codes and descriptions found in this subsection illustrate the method used to test (e.g., automated, non-automated, dip stick, with or without microscopy), kind of substance (e.g., ketones) for (e.g., qualitative), the color of the specimen and the amount (volume). If you are trying to test for a particular substance (e.g., if you want to find out if a woman is pregnant and you test for human chorionic gonadotropin in the urine), you should use the codes under other subsections (e.g., chemistry – see 84702/84703 for HCG).

As we have explained in the beginning of this chapter on Pathology and Laboratory, there are many sections within which the descriptions are arranged alphabetically. The Chemistry subsection is one of these.

What is unique here in the Chemistry subsection is that you are testing for the chemical components found in these specimens. When you look at these codes, you will see that the specimens can come from any source. That is, you may be testing for something using urine, blood, saliva, etc.

For example:

82000 *Acetaldehyde, blood*

or

82106 *Alpha-fetoprotein; amniotic fluid*

Note that in both of these examples, the test was for a special component found in a particular kind of specimen.

There may be instances in which you are testing for several analytes that come from a specimen. In these cases, it is appropriate to use the codes that are applicable to code for all of the services you provide given that the substances are not already part of the description of the code.

For example, if you were testing a patient for both ammonia and albumin in the urine, you could use the code 82140 for the ammonia test and 82042 for the albumin test.

The majority of the tests found in the Chemistry subsection are considered to be quantitative. That is, the measurement is to discover whether a substance is present. Unless the code says otherwise, the *amount* of a substance that is present in a particular specimen is not reported using these codes.

There are some codes that bear special consideration and explanation (see codes 82491 – 82492 and 82541- 82544). These are the ones that include the measurement of several substances by various methods that are all in one code. For instance, consider the following.

82492 *Chromatography, quantitative, column (e.g., liquid or HPLC); multiple analytes, single stationary and mobile phase*

As you can see by reading the description of this code, you may be testing multiple substances *and* these might be tested using both the single stationary *and* mobile phases.

What if however, you were testing multiple analytes, some using the stationary phase and others using the mobile phase. Since the code describes the use of multiple analytes using BOTH the stationary

AND mobile phases, the use of the one code number, 82492, would be sufficient to describe both phases of the analytes.

The importance of reading and rereading code descriptions to pick up on nuances like this cannot be overstated.

Hematology

Again you will see that the arrangement of the code descriptions is alphabetical. Following are some of the kinds of things tested here:

a. bleeding times
b. blood counts
c. blood smears
d. bone marrows
e. clotting
f. fibrin, fibrinogen, fibrinolysins
g. platelets
h. thrombin time, thromboplastin, etc.

Note that there are specific words included in the descriptions that help identify particularities of a test. For example, portions of the description for the blood count may be repeated from one code to the other, but when you read the description in its entirety, you learn about the specific differences in each code.

For example:

85025 *Blood count; complete (CBC), automated (Hgb, Hct, RBC, WBC and platelet count) and automated differential WBC*

85027 *Blood count; complete (CBC), automated (Hgb, Hct, RBC, WBC and platelet count)*

Once you know the specifics of what test(s) was (were) actually provided, you can weed out the portions that do not apply (from code to code) and pick the one(s) that include(s) the actual test(s) you provided.

You will see that the codes for obtaining bone marrow aspiration and bone marrow biopsy are referenced here but that you are sent to the Surgery section to actually get the correct code for the obtaining of the specimen (e.g., the **CPT** book tells you to go to codes 38220, 38221, 20220, 20225, 20240, 20245, 20250, 20251, 38230, and 38240). Sending you to the Surgery Section is appropriate as the procedure to obtain the specimen is an invasive one and belongs in the invasive (Surgery) section.

Cytopathology

Let's suppose that you work at a family practice office and one of your patients comes in for her annual physical. You complete the history and exam, find no problems of any significance and also take a routine Pap smear. You would code this Pap smear using the number 88150, which simply states that you provided cytopathology, slides of the cervix or vagina Note that this code implies that your physician's assistant or nurse could have taken the smear. Also note that there are a variety of combinations of this code that are almost extension like, giving you other options for coding the smear if a computer re-screening were done or combinations of this idea thereof. Now, if the Pap smear required the interpretation by the physician (or pathologist), you would also need to report another code, 88141, in addition to the code for the obtaining of the specimen which states the following:

+88141 *Cytopathology, cervical or vaginal (any reporting system); requiring interpretation by physician (list separately in addition to code for technical service)*

Notice that this code specifically tells you to use it in addition to the code for the slide when the interpretive services of the physician are required.

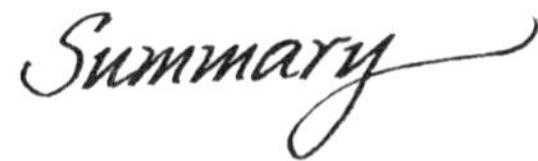

CHAPTER NINE

- ✔ Codes found in the Pathology and Laboratory Section begin with the number 8.

- ✔ It is important to read and understand all information found in the subsection "notes," as well as any information in parentheses.

- ✔ In submitting an unlisted procedure or a procedure with modifier -22, Unusual Service, it is important that you include a special written report that can be understood by the average layperson.

- ✔ In coding for tests in the Organ or Disease-Oriented Panels, you must make sure that the panel you choose includes the complete list of tests described under each one.

- ✔ Any tests not included in the list of tests for each panel should be reported separately and in addition to the other service(s).

✔ There are different kinds of consultations that are identified within the Pathology and Laboratory Section. These include consultations on slides made elsewhere, consultations on specimens requiring you to make slides and consultations made during surgery.

✔ Some Surgical Pathology codes are divided into levels. The level of a given specimen depends on the degree of difficulty involved in the physician's evaluation of that specimen (e.g., higher levels are associated with greater degrees of pathology), as well as where the specimen came from (for example, cervix vs. colon).

✔ Be sure to read the different specimen listings under each code in the Surgical Pathology subsection. Remember that the same specimen may be mentioned in several different codes throughout this subsection. By carefully reading each code description you will be able to select the code that most closely describes the services you performed.

CHAPTER TEN

MEDICINE

Codes in Medicine, the last major section of **CPT**, begin with the number 9. Placement of this section at the end of the book allows all of the chapters to be in numerical order (except for the Evaluation and Management Section, the first major section, whose codes also begin with 9).

Editorial notations found in the Medicine Section are the bullet (●) for new codes, the triangle (▲) for revised descriptors, the inverted triangles (▸ ◂) for new/revised text around the codes, add-on codes(✚) for like supplemental services in addition to the primary procedure, and the exempt sign (⃠) for codes that are "exempt" from the use of the multiple service modifier - 51. No starred codes are found in the Medicine Section; they are found only after codes in the Surgery Section, which begin with the numbers 1, 2, 3, 4, 5, and 6.

IMMUNIZATIONS: IMMUNE GLOBULINS AND IMMUNIZATIONS ADMINISTRATION FOR VACCINES/TOXOIDS

The Immunization and Immune Globulins subsection found in the Medicine Section changed significantly in 1999. You will see that **CPT** divides these subsections (codes 90281 through 90749) into the following sub-subsections.

These include:

- Immune Globulins
- Immunization Administration for Vaccines/Toxoids
- Vaccines, Toxoids

Let us look at some of the peculiarities of the codes in this subsection. To begin with, the codes found here include either the vaccine only or the administration of the vaccine *but not both.* That is, there is the process of injecting the vaccine which is different than the supply of the vaccine itself. Because of this, you will

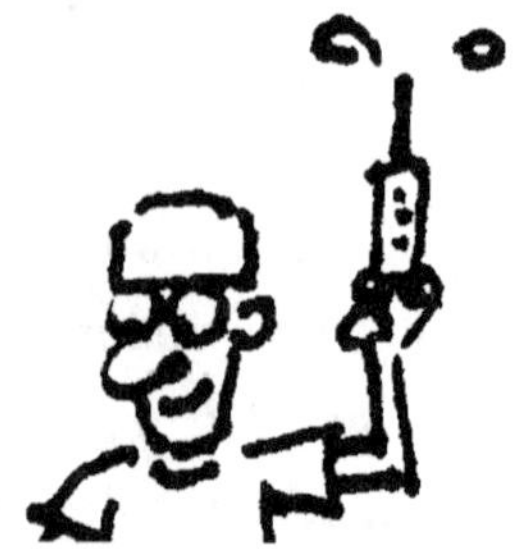

Are you ready?

need to code for (and bill) a number for the material injected and one for the *process of* giving the drug. Remember to code for both the supply and the administration.

Consider what would happen if a mother brought her four year-old child in for a tetanus toxoid injection during which no other services were performed. You would code this in the following way:

90471 *Immunization administration (includes percutaneous, intradermal, subcutaneous, intramuscular and jet injections); one vaccine (single or combination vaccine/ toxoid)*

90703 *Tetanus toxoid absorbed, for intramuscular or jet injection use*

Note that the codes 90471 and 90703 must be used together. You cannot use the administration code 90471 and not show what you administered (e.g., 90703).

As **CPT** explains, however, immunization injections usually are given when the patient is receiving other services from the physician (e.g., regular yearly physical-gynecological exam). When an immunization injection is given at the time of such a visit, **CPT** says to code the service (usually an E/M service, see 99201 through 99215), the supply of material injected, and the actual administration of the immunization.

This is an example of how the coding would appear:

99202 *Office or other outpatient visit for the evaluation and management of a new patient, which requires these three key components:*

- *a detailed history;*
- *a detailed exam; and*
- *medical decision-making of low complexity*

Counseling and/or coordination of care with other providers or agencies are provided consistent with the nature of the problem(s) and the patient's and/or family's needs.

Usually the presenting problem(s) are of moderate severity.

Physicians typically spend 20 minutes face-to-face with the patient or family.

90471 *Immunization administration (includes percutaneous, intradermal, subcutaneous, intramuscular and jet injections); one vaccine (single or combination vaccine/ toxoid)*

90713 *Poliovirus vaccine, inactivated, (IPV), for subcutaneous use*

For each of these services, the coder would list a price. Claim forms from hundreds of offices have shown that many coders bill only for the immunization injection and forget (or don't know about) coding for the visit that accompanied it, or they don't realize that the coding rules have changed, and therefore, they forget to bill separately for the drug or component injected as well as the procedure of injecting.

THERAPEUTIC OR DIAGNOSTIC INJECTIONS

For therapeutic or diagnostic injections (codes 90782 through 90799), the rules differ somewhat from those of immunization injections.

When you look at the codes for injections, you will note that you are asked to specify **what** was injected. Let's look at a typical therapeutic injection code:

90782 *Therapeutic, prophylactic or diagnostic injection (specify material injected); subcutaneous or intramuscular*

As you can see from the above, the coder is requested to specify the substance injected subcutaneously or intramuscularly. The following is a list of some possibilities:

- *cortisone, up to 50 mg;*
- *depo-medrol, 40 mg;*
- *depo-medrol, 80 mg;*
- *estrogen, conjugated up to 2 mg;*
- *gold sodium thiosulfate, up to 50 mg.*

Using **CPT**, what code number would you select for the coding of these injections? You probably would choose 90782, because all of these substances are given subcutaneously or intramuscularly. This would be the correct code if you were using only **CPT.**

Having selected 90782 for the coding of these therapeutic injections, let's fill in the "specify" part as the description of 90782 requests.

Code	Description	Fee
90782	*Therapeutic, prophylactic or diagnostic injection (cortisone, 50 mg); subcutaneous or intramuscular*	*$ 2.00**
90782	*Therapeutic, prophylactic or diagnostic injection (depo-medrol = methyl prednisolone acetate, 40 mg); subcutaneous or intramuscular*	*$10.00**
90782	*Therapeutic, prophylactic or diagnostic injection (depo-medrol = methyl prednisolone acetate, 80 mg); subcutaneous or intramuscular*	*$19.50**
90782	*Therapeutic, prophylactic or diagnostic injection (estrogen, conjugated up to 2 mg); subcutaneous or intramuscular*	*$28.00**
90782	*Therapeutic, prophylactic or diagnostic injection (gold sodium thiosulfate, up to 50 mg);subcutaneous or intramuscular*	*$50.00**

*The fees listed here are fictitious and should not be assumed by the reader to be real or suggested fees. They are printed here only for use in this example.

As you can see by comparing the prices of the injectable substances above, the prices vary, yet the code 90782 remains constant.

Furthermore, when your claim is entered into the computer at any insurance company or even if you submit your claims electronically, there is no way to communicate to the computer (other than through the code choices you make) about any nuances that may apply to a particular code. The computer reads **CPT** codes--that's why you use them. Because the computer does not read the code description, you must find a way to distinguish among the different kinds of drugs or injectables that may be supplied. Why? Because since the current HCFA 1500 claim form has no space for a description of the items given, using a unique code for a particular substance is the only way you can communicate to the computer at the insurance company about the differences in the substances that were injected and let them know that each of them had its own unique cost.

Differentiating among the kinds of substances injected is easy when you use the **National Coding Manual**. If you recall, all injections are listed under the J section for injections.

Looking up these substances in the **National Coding Manual**, you may find the following:

J0287 *Injection, Amphotericin B Lipid Complex, 10 mg* *

J1030 *Injection, methylprednisolone acetate, 40 mg* *

J1040 *Injection, methylprednisolone acetate, 80 mg* *

J1410 *Injection, estrogen conjugated, per 25 mg* *

J1600 *Injection, gold sodium thiomalate, up to 50 mg* *

*These codes were taken from the 2003 Official Medicare version of the **HCPCS National Coding Manual**.

As you can see, the description of each substance is represented by a different **J** code. This way, the computer can recognize the substance for which it must reimburse by recognizing the distinct code number.

PSYCHIATRY

The section on Psychiatry is listed in the Medicine Section because in most cases, the psychiatrist is not performing physical exams, which are an inherent part of the majority of Evaluation and Management codes. A psychiatrist may use the Evaluation and Management service codes if he/she provides the key components (history, exam and medical decision-making) that are part of the Evaluation and Management codes. An example of this would be when the physician sees a patient in the hospital and must write orders, discuss therapy with the nurses, order tests, etc. In this case, the use of the appropriate Evaluation and Management code is appropriate.

Let's take a look at an example of a psychiatry code.

90804 *Individual psychotherapy, insight-oriented, behavior modifying and/or supportive, in an office or outpatient facility, approximately 20 to 30 minutes face-to-face with the patient;*

90805	*with medical evaluation and management services*
90806	*Individual psychotherapy, insight-oriented, behavior modifying and/or supportive, in an office or outpatient facility, approximately 45 to 50 minutes face-to-face with the patient;*
90807	*with medical evaluation and management services*

You can see two things from these codes. The first is that if you provided medical evaluation and management, you have the option with these codes of selecting one of the code numbers (i.e., 90805 or 90807) that includes the medical evaluation and management (see actual descriptions of codes listed above). The other thing that you will notice is that all of the services (90804 through 90807) list references to an amount of time spent with the patient. This is very common in the Psychiatry subsection as the treatment is usually consultative in nature and requires the physician to talk things out with the patient. Some patients may take longer than others due to the nature of their issues and **CPT** makes the provision of giving different times frames within the different codes to allow for these differences.

Interactive Psychotherapy versus Insight-Oriented, Behavior Modifying and/or Supportive Psychotherapy

The **CPT** book makes a clear distinction about the different kinds of therapy that a physician can provide by giving the coder two different sections of codes to choose from. Each of these sections specifies, within a particular code in the section, exact amounts of time that the physician spends with the patient. The first of these subsections, Insight-Oriented, Behavior Modifying and/or Supportive Psychotherapy, is generally used on adults or those individuals who are able to articulate to the physician what their problems or concerns may be. In these situations, the physician can talk with the patient and gain some semblance of what the issues are. In some situations, however (e.g., with children), it is more difficult for the physician to get a grasp on the issues. The Interactive Psychotherapy subsection helps the coder by providing codes that include play therapy or the use of toys or other physical aids that help the clinician gain some insight as to the problems. These aids can also help the physician communicate with the patient.

You can also see by the heading preceding the subsection beginning with the code 90804 that the **CPT** book makes a distinction between those psychiatry services provided in an office or other outpatient facility and the inpatient hospital, partial hospital or residential care facility. Make sure that you know *where* the service occurred (inpatient or office/outpatient), *how* it occurred (play therapy or interactive), the *amount of time* that the physician spent with the patient, and if any other services were provided at the same date (e.g., Evaluation and Management services, electroconvulsive therapy). Only then will you have enough information to correctly code for the procedure.

Finally, check out the subsections on Other Psychotherapy and Other Psychiatric Services or Procedures. You will find codes there that describe services such as multiple-family group psychotherapy, group psychotherapy (other than multiple family), preparation of reports for legal or consultative purposes, or for insurance companies, other physicians, etc., hypnotherapy, pharmacologic management, etc. All of these codes are self-explanatory and merit your reading in the **CPT** book.

You will also find some codes for Central Nervous System assessments and tests (e.g., psychological testing that includes psychodiagnostic assessment of personality, psychopathology, emotionality and intellectual abilities (see 96100 through 96117) and health and behavior assessment/intervention (see 96150 through 96155)). Make sure that you take a look at these codes if you are providing these kinds of services.

DIALYSIS

The Dialysis subsection in **CPT** is short and to the point. It describes services that are done by the month (see codes 90918 through 90921) or per day (90922 through 90925). Similar in concept to the Preventive Medicine codes we saw in the Evaluation and Management Section, these codes are differentiated based upon the age of the patient. For example, the difference between the codes 90922 and 90923 is that in the 90922, the patient is under two years of age and in the 90923, the patient is between two and eleven years of age.

It is important to note that the per month codes include the normal care (not requiring any hospitalization during the month), including establishment of the patient's regimen for dialysis, the evaluation and management that goes along with the dialysis sessions, any necessary phone calls and any patient management that happens during the treatments. These per month visits do NOT include the "dialysis" itself or anything else not listed above. Dialysis services would be reported using the codes 90935, 90937, 90945 and 90947.

GASTROENTEROLOGY

Like many other codes and subsections found in the **CPT** book, the Gastroenterology subsection has a variety of codes and descriptions for things like esophageal intubation for obtaining washings, gastric motility studies, gastric intubations, anal manometry, irrigation of fecal impaction, etc. Although in some of these instances there are devices placed inside the patient's body (e.g., intubations or irrigations for fecal impaction), the services are not considered "invasive" enough to place them in the surgery section. When choosing a code from this subsection, make sure to read all of the possibilities that may apply so that you can select the code as accurately as possible.

OPHTHALMOLOGY

You will notice that there is a special subsection of the Medicine Chapter dedicated to Ophthalmologic services. And, when you look at these services, you will see that they are, for the ophthalmologist, the Evaluation and Management services that are unique to the ophthalmology profession. One would argue these codes are not placed in the Evaluation and Management Section because they are so specialized (just as there are other unique subsections for other specialties found within the Medicine Section of **CPT**, e.g., gastroenterology, dialysis, psychiatry) and that many of these Ophthalmology codes include services that go beyond the key components (history, exam and medical decision-making) found in the routine Evaluation and Management services.

To that end, you will note several nuances of the Ophthalmology subsection that bear special consideration. First, the services listed in the Ophthalmology Section are considered to be bilateral. That is, the services include both eyes. When you examine one eye, it is "understood" that you will also examine the other. When you only examine one eye, the addition of a modifier to the service code will be necessary to indicate that the service was reduced or partially eliminated. The modifier -52 indicates Reduced Services, and we will discuss it more in the chapter on modifiers (see Chapter Eleven).

Another issue of special significance in the Ophthalmology subsection is that there are only two "levels" of service that one will find for new and established patients (see 92002 and 92004 for new patients and 92012 and 92014 for established patients). The definitions for new and established patient are the same in the Medicine Section as in the Evaluation and Management Section. That is, a new patient is one who is new to the physician and who has not received any face-to-face professional services from the physician in the past three years. An established patient is one who has received face-to-face professional services from the physician in the past three years. Each of these services for both new and established patients (no matter the "level") includes the following components:

- *slit lamp exam;*
- *keratometry;*
- *routine ophthalmoscopy;*
- *retinoscopy;*
- *tonometry;*
- *motor evaluation.*

Put another way, each of the office type visits (92002, 92004, 92012, 92014) includes as many of the services listed above as are applicable for a particular physician/patient encounter.

You will notice that the determination of the refractive state is not listed as part of the group above. The determination of the refractive state (92015) can be found in the Special Ophthalmological Services subsection and should be reported in addition to the code for the visit.

Let us now discuss what some of the terminology in this subsection means and how you will go about using the numbers here. You will find the word "intermediate" used in codes 92002 and 92102. This word denotes that the physician provided a history, general medical observation, external ocular and adnexal examination and other diagnostic services listed above (as the patient may need), possibly including the use of mydriasis for ophthalmoscopy. The codes describe a situation in which the regular Evaluation and Management service doesn't apply (even though you are still providing some sort of history, exam and medical decision-making and even though it may apply to either a new condition or an existing condition complicated with a new problem) because you are providing the other additional services (see above) that are not included with a regular E/M service. The code also describes a situation in which you do not have to make an inspection of the complete visual system.

A comprehensive exam (see code 92004 and 92014) takes into account the services rendered to inspect the complete visual system. Additionally, the service includes obtaining the patient's history (if applicable), a general medical observation, both external and ophthalmologic exams, gross visual fields and a basic sensorimotor exam. A comprehensive exam could also include biomicroscopy, examination with cycloplegia or mydriasis and tonometry. It always includes the initiation of diagnostic and treatment programs. The comprehensive exam does not include the determination of the refractive state.

Many coders for ophthalmology miss the boat by assuming that since the prescription of glasses is an inherent part of the general ophthalmologic service (it is included in the determination of the refractive state which is part of the regular visit), that the prescription for contacts is the same. This is not true. When contacts are prescribed, a separate code (see 92310 through 92326) should be employed.

Let's take some examples. Suppose an established patient comes to your clinic for her regular eye exam. Your technician performs both the external and ophthalmoscopic exams and the gross visual fields, does a basic sensorimotor exam and asks to see the patient's glasses. During the visit, the patient reports that her vision has gotten worse over the past year. The technician determines the refractive state, notes that the patient is not aphakic, and jots down his findings for the physician. The physician reviews the notes taken by the technician and questions the patient about her condition. During the visit, the physician concludes that the patient needs new glasses and reviews the determination of the refractive state performed by the technician.

The coding you would use to describe this would be the following:

92014 *Ophthalmologic services: medical examination and evaluation, with initiation or continuation of diagnostic and treatment program; comprehensive, established patient one or more visits*

92015 *Determination of the refractive state*

Let's say that another patient comes to your office and the exact same service happens, only at this visit, the patient decides that he wants to have contacts in addition to the glasses. The physician completes the prescription and fitting of the contacts and codes for the following:

92014	*Ophthalmologic services: medical examination and evaluation, with initiation or continuation of diagnostic and treatment program; comprehensive, established patient one or more visits*
92015	*Determination of the refractive state*
92310	*Prescription of optical and physical characteristics of and fitting of contact lens, with medical supervision of adaptation; corneal lens, both eyes, except aphakia*

Note how there is an "extra" code for the prescription of the contacts that is separate and in addition to the other codes that were used.

There are also some codes that apply to ophthalmology type services in the back of the Medicine Section (see codes 99172 and 99173). These codes pertain to visual function screening and screening of visual acuity. Why these codes are not part of the Ophthalmology subsection is unclear. If you are providing these kinds of services, make sure to check out this portion of your **CPT** book.

Finally, there is a special supply section found under this Ophthalmology subsection. It is unique in that there are few, if other specialties that have their own subsection for supplies. It is here that you will find codes for the supply of spectacles, contacts, low vision aids, ocular prostheses, etc. Keep in mind that you may also find these same supplies (and more) in the **HCPCS National Coding Manual**.

SPECIAL OTORHINOLARYNGOLOGIC SERVICES

There are many services that an otorhinolaryngologist (ENT guy) may perform that would be normal parts of the comprehensive type of Evaluation and Management service done by this specialist (e.g., otoscopy, rhinoscopy, tuning fork or whispered fork tests). When the physician does these services during the regular Evaluation and Management visit, you will not need to report them separately (i.e., they are already included). But, when the services are not part of these routine-type services, you will need to code them separately.

In this subsection of Medicine, you will find services that are both non-invasive and/or diagnostic and that are *not* included in the regular Evaluation and Management services performed by the physician during the normal doctor-patient encounter. These procedures include services like nasal function studies (92512) or aural rehabilitation (92510), which can be coded in addition to the Evaluation and Management codes when performed at the same time. You will also see services such as vestibular function tests and audiologic function tests that can be coded in *addition to* the codes for the Evaluation and Management services when performed at the same encounter.

Use of the codes in the Special Otorhinolaryngologic subsection implies that the physician is testing both ears. There are, however, instances when the physician will only test one ear. When this happens, you will need to use a modifier to explain to the computer at the carrier's office that only one ear was tested. The modifier that you will employ is the modifier -52, Reduced Services. We will discuss this modifier in more detail in Chapter Eleven, Modifiers.

In 2003, a special subsection was added to Medicine for Evaluative and Therapeutic services for ENT. These procedures include (but are not limited to) diagnostic analysis of cochlear implants (see 92601- 92604), services for both speech generating augmentative and alternative and non-speech generating augmentative and alternative devices (see 95605 through 92609), evaluations of swallowing function (see 92610 through92613) and endoscopic examinations (92614 though 92617).

With regard to the analysis of the cochlear implants keep in mind that these services are provided postoperatively.

Let's say that a patient who is 8 comes to your office with his grandmother because the patient has been deaf all their life and the grandmother heard on the local public broadcasting station about cochlear implants. Your physician placed the cochlear implant several months ago and the patient is returning for an analyses of the device. You examine the patient's device and re-program the external transmitter to better meet the patient's needs. You would code this in the following way.

92604 *Diagnostic analysis of cochlear implant, age 7 years or older; subsequent reprogramming*

Note that the code you picked describes three things in this example. First, the code implies that the service occurred after the surgery (postoperatively) although how far away from the surgery date, we do not know. Second, the code implies that the age of the patient is at least 7 (but could be more) based upon what the description of the code says. If your patient was under the age of 7, you would need to pick another code. Last but not least, the description tells you that the external transmitter was re-programmed.

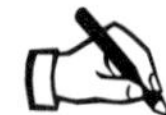

Remember: "Make sure that you read and re-read all of the information in and around the codes so that you can pick the most accurate code possible.

CARDIOVASCULAR

The cardiovascular subsection of Medicine is extensive. Reviewing it, you will see the following:

- *Therapeutic Services*
- *Cardiography*
- *Echocardiogarphy*
- *Cardiac Catherization*
- *Repair of septal defects*
- *Intracardiac Electrophysiological Procedures/Studies*
- *Peripheral Arterial Disease Rehabilitation*

- *Other Vascular Studies*
- *Other Procedures*

As you can see by looking at these subsections, most of the codes found here are either non-invasive or diagnostic in nature (e.g., cardiac catherization includes the introduction of the catheter, the positioning and possibly the repositioning of the catheter, the recording of intracardiac and intravascular pressure and the obtaining of blood samples). These codes are found in the Medicine Section (as opposed to the Surgery Section when they appear to be invasive) because the invasive nature of these services does not include cutting on anyone, replacing or repairing anything or taking anything out (as we see in Surgery).

There are some codes in the Medicine Section for catheter closure of an atreal septal defect (93580) and for catheter closure of a ventricular septal defect (93581). While both of these codes appear to be "*invasive*" and one would suppose that they should be placed in the Surgery Section, they were placed in the Medicine Section because they are performed by an interventional cardiologist (someone who works to alter the course of disease or improve the health of the patient).

You will see in the Cardiovascular subsection that there are some add-on codes. As you will recall, add-on codes can go together with other services at the same session. Let's look at an example.

Suppose a patient presents for a comprehensive electrophysiologic evaluation with right arterial pacing and recording, right ventricular pacing and recording, Bundle of His recording, with insertion of multiple electrode catheters in an attempt to induce an arrhythmia, and your physician also performs the same services on the patient's left. You would code the entire procedure using the following codes:

93620 *Comprehensive electrophysiologic evaluation including insertion and repositioning of multiple electrode catheters with introduction or attempted introduction of arrhythmia; with right atrial pacing and recording, right ventricular pacing and recording, His bundle recording*

93621 *with left atrial pacing and recording from coronary sinus or left atrium*

+93622 *with left ventricular pacing and recording*

Although it is not necessary to add the plus signs (+) to the codes when you actually place the numbers on the HCFA 1500 claim form, it is important for you to get the idea that the plus sign means that you can continue to add on as many codes as necessary to completely show any carrier what services were provided to the patient.

ALLERGY AND CLINICAL IMMUNOLOGY

You will notice that the Allergy subsection includes two different types of services that are independent of and not immediately related to any Evaluation and Management services. The services found here include both the testing of the patient and the treatment of the patient with immunotherapy.

ALLERGY TESTING

In this subsection you will note that there are many different kinds of allergy tests that can be administered. These include percutaneous tests, skin end point titrations, patch or application tests, ophthalmic mucous membrane tests, direct nasal mucous tests and others. To use many of these codes correctly, the description of the code asks that you specify the number of the tests performed. For example, let's say that a patient came in and received the percutaneous type tests with allergenic extracts to tests for five different allergies. You would select the code 95004, which describes the appropriate kind of tests, but you would need to specify the number of tests performed (in this case 5) in the units column (see Space 24G) of the HCFA 1500 claim form.

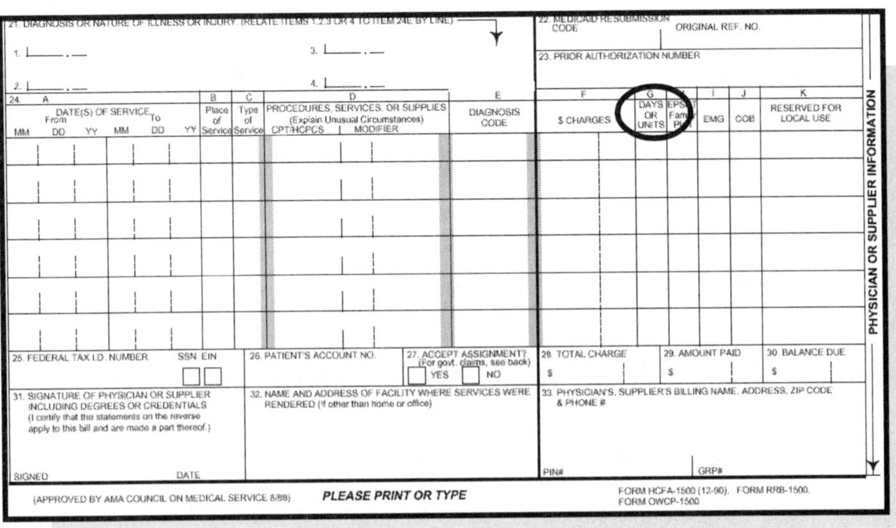

21. DIAGNOSIS OR NATURE OF ILLNESS OR INJURY. (RELATE ITEMS 1,2,3 OR 4 TO ITEM 24E BY LINE)

1. ___ . __
2. ___ . __
3. ___ . __
4. ___ . __

22. MEDICAID RESUBMISSION CODE | ORIGINAL REF. NO.

23. PRIOR AUTHORIZATION NUMBER

24. A DATE(S) OF SERVICE From MM DD YY To MM DD YY	B Place of Service	C Type of Service	D PROCEDURES, SERVICES, OR SUPPLIES (Explain Unusual Circumstances) CPT/HCPCS | MODIFIER	E DIAGNOSIS CODE	F $ CHARGES	G DAYS OR UNITS	H EPSDT Family Plan	I EMG	J COB	K RESERVED FOR LOCAL USE

PHYSICIAN OR SUPPLIER INFORMATION

25. FEDERAL TAX I.D. NUMBER SSN EIN

26. PATIENT'S ACCOUNT NO.

27. ACCEPT ASSIGNMENT? (For govt. claims, see back) YES NO

28. TOTAL CHARGE $

29. AMOUNT PAID $

30. BALANCE DUE $

31. SIGNATURE OF PHYSICIAN OR SUPPLIER INCLUDING DEGREES OR CREDENTIALS (I certify that the statements on the reverse apply to this bill and are made a part thereof.)

SIGNED DATE

32. NAME AND ADDRESS OF FACILITY WHERE SERVICES WERE RENDERED (If other than home or office)

33. PHYSICIAN'S, SUPPLIER'S BILLING NAME, ADDRESS, ZIP CODE & PHONE #

PIN# GRP#

(APPROVED BY AMA COUNCIL ON MEDICAL SERVICE 8/88) **PLEASE PRINT OR TYPE** FORM HCFA-1500 (12-90), FORM RRB-1500, FORM OWCP-1500

The placement of the number 5 in this space indicates to the insurance company that five tests were provided to the patient. More information about the use of the HCFA 1500 claim form and how to complete it will be given to you in Chapter Twelve.

Many coders lose money either for their offices or for the patients because they do not thoroughly read the descriptions of the codes and use them as indicated. Make sure that you are not one of these coders and that you take the time to specify the number of tests.

Once the patient has been properly diagnosed and you begin treatment, you will need to make note of another nuance. Within the Allergen Immunotherapy subsection, you will find two different kinds of codes. The first set (95115 through 95134) includes those in which the physician does not provide the allergenic extracts (e.g., the physician or his or her staff simply administers the shot), and the second set of codes (95144 through 95170) actually includes the provision of the antigen. Make sure that you find out which of these your office actually did before employing a specific code.

Chemotherapy Injections

According to **CPT**, the injection of a chemotherapeutic agent (code numbers 96400 through 96549) is independent of the patient's visit. In plain English, whether the injection was administered on the same day of the visit or afterward doesn't matter; these injections are still billed separately.

According to the rules implemented by CMS, because cancer chemotherapy injections are more complex than other kinds of injections, Medicare will pay for all injection procedures in this range of codes separate from and in addition to any visit or service rendered on the same or a different day.

PHYSICAL MEDICINE AND REHABILITATION

There has been a lot of abuse of the subsection on Physical Medicine and Rehabilitation. Let's discuss how this can happen. As you can see by looking at this subsection, some of the services can be "supervised" while others require that the therapist be in "constant attention". Supervised services mean that the therapist can come and go as he or she pleases, making sure that the patient is taken care of and making sure to check in with the patient to see how things are going. Supervised services do not require that the therapist be one-on-one with the patient for the entire time. In contrast, "constant attendance" requires that the therapist be with the patient one-on-one for the entire visit.

Some not so scrupulous groups will code for services that require constant attention even though they do not provide it. Not only is this unethical, if discovered by either a patient or insurance company, huge sanctions can apply.

You will note that the supervised modalities (codes 97010 through 97028) are very specific about what is applied to the patient. For example, consider the following:

97012 Application of a modality to one or more areas; traction, mechanical

As you can see, by using the word "traction," the book specifically tells the coder that two parts must be pulled away from each other. The word "mechanical" implies that the traction itself or the pulling was provided by a device rather than an individual. Once again, it cannot be overstated that reading and understanding what is and is not included in each code description is critical to proper and effective coding.

You will also note that within both the Constant Attendance and Therapeutic Procedures subsections of Physical Medicine and Rehabilitation, the codes list time frames for the respective services. Usually the time frames are given in 15-minute increments. If you provided services for more than the specified 15 minutes, you would need to indicate that by placing the quantity of 15-minute increments in the units column of the HCFA 1500 claim form (as we talked about under Allergy and Clinical Immunology).

OTHER SUBSECTIONS OF THE MEDICINE SECTION

For most general coders, the balance of the Medicine Section contains codes for noninvasive procedures such as the following:

- Biofeedback
- Gastroenterology
- Noninvasive vascular diagnostic studies
- Pulmonary
- Endocrinology
- Neurology and neuromuscular procedures
- Central nervous system assessments/tests
- Special dermatological procedures
- Medical nutrition therapy
- Osteopathic manipulative treatment
- Chiropractic
- Qualifying circumstances for anesthesia
- Sedation with or without analgesia
- Other services

Since none of these procedures involves cutting anyone open or taking anything out, they are deemed non-invasive.

It is good to remember that specialties may have different procedures listed in different sections of **CPT**. For example, *non*invasive dermatologic procedures (e.g., actinotherapy treatment with ultraviolet light) are listed in the Medicine Section and invasive dermatologic procedures (e.g., incision and drainage) in the Surgery Section. *Non*invasive ophthalmologic procedures (e.g., determination of the refractive state) are listed in the Medicine Section and invasive ophthalmologic procedures (e.g., cataract surgeries) in the Surgery Section.

Once you determine whether a procedure is invasive or noninvasive, you will have a much easier time locating the section in which the code can be found.

Special Services And Reports

Special Services and Reports is a subsection found at the end of the Medicine section in the range of codes from 99000 to 99091. Although many coders are unaware of this subsection or don't know how to use it properly, it is certainly one of the most interesting sections of **CPT**.

As you can see by the first paragraph in the heading of this subsection, codes 99000 (handling of a specimen) through 99091 (collection and interpretation of physiologic data) are *adjunct* codes to basic services rendered (you *add* them to the other *junk* you do: adjunct). In other words, they should be added to the claim with other codes in order to completely delineate the service(s) provided. Let's examine these codes in detail and look at examples of their use by the coder in completing claim forms.

Specimen Handling

99000 *Handling and/or conveyance of a specimen for transfer from the physician's office to a laboratory*

Use of the 99000 code is indicated when the coder wants to show that some specimen (such as blood, urine, or a biopsy) was collected in the physician's office, handled there (e.g., centrifuged), and then sent to a lab. Up to and including year 1984, 99000 was used to code for both collection and handling of specimens. The collection part was deleted from this code in 1985 because not all specimens (e.g., urine samples) were collected by physicians. When the specimen was, in fact, collected by a physician, the act of collecting the specimen was billed separately. For examples, look up 36415* for collection of blood, and other appropriate codes for biopsies performed in your office. (Note: The stars or asterisks on codes like 36415 apply to rules on Starred Procedures, which are discussed in the Surgery Chapter.)

99001 *Handling and/or conveyance of specimen for transfer from the patient, in other than a physician's office, to a laboratory (distance may be indicated)*

The use of 99001 is indicated when the coder wants to show that a specimen, collected in some place other than the physician's office, was sent to a lab. Examples are the transfer of a specimen from a nursing home to a lab and from the patient's home to a lab.

99002 *Handling, conveyance, and/or any other service in connection with the implementation of an order involving devices (e.g., designing, fitting, packaging, handling, delivery, or mailing)when devices such as orthotics, protectives, or prosthetics are fabricated by an outside laboratory or shop but which items have been designed, and are to be fitted and adjusted, by the attending physician*

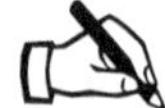

Remember: If the patient does the handling or transferring of a specimen or device, you should not be billing for this procedure.

As a handling code, how does 99002 differ from 99000 and 99001?

Code 99002 should be used for the handling of a **device** (e.g., an artificial limb or brace, an artificial eye, or anything that has to be designed and fitted by the attending physician). You will notice that everything is included in this number: charges for the mailing service, cost of the packaging (styrofoam peanuts, scotch tape, cardboard box, etc.), and handling charges.

The other two handling codes, 99000 and 99001, are used for specimens **only,** not devices.

POSTOPERATIVE FOLLOW-UP VISITS

99024 Postoperative follow-up visit, included in global service

You may use this code to indicate visits from a patient following surgery.

Many patients submit all of their insurance claim forms, whether or not the services are to be reimbursed. Patients may not realize that you haven't placed a charge on the form, and will submit the claim. To code for follow-up visits included in the Surgical

Package on claim forms that patients may submit, use code 99024 and "N/C" for "no charge." If you place "N/C" next to an office visit code for a postoperative visit, and if this patient turns in the claim form, the "N/C" charge could be entered as a $0 with other charges you normally make for that office visit code. Instead of using an office visit code, use code 99024.

The use of the 99024 accurately reports the kind of service (the re-check) that was performed postoperatively.

Visit Codes for Starred Procedures

99025 *Initial (new patient) visit when starred (*) surgical procedure constitutes major service at that visit*

This code is explained in detail in the Surgery Chapter. As you may recall, it should be used when a relatively small surgical procedure (e.g., venipuncture or blood draw) is performed on a patient who is new to your office and for whom this starred procedure was the major service provided at that visit.

The next two codes, 99026 and 99027 were new to the **CPT** book in 2003. Let's take a look at them below.

99026 *Hospital mandated on call service; in hospital, each hour*

99027 *out-of-hospital, each hour*

Because these codes fall in between 99000 and 99091 they are also considered to be adjunct codes. You can use them when you are on call (as required by the hospital) and you are called to the hospital to render a service. For example, suppose you are the physician on call (as required by the hospital) and the emergency room calls you to tell you that there is a patient there who has been in a severe car accident and who needs to go to surgery for repair of severe gashes to the abdominal area. You go to the hospital and wait for about 10 minutes until the life flight helicopter arrives so that you can perform surgery. When the patient arrives, you complete your assessment, ask some questions of the paramedics and proceed to remove the patient's right kidney and spleen. Not only would you code for the emergency room assessment (using the correct modifier showing that this service was where the decision to operate was made, see modifier –57), but you would also code for the removal of the kidney and spleen, and for the 99027 as you were out of the hospital and were called to provide the "on call" services. If you had to standby for a long period of time, you may want to also consider the use of the code 99360.

ADJUNCT CODES

As we have already stated, codes 99000 through 99091 are adjunct codes. That is, they are used **in addition to** codes that describe other procedures or services your physician performs. For example, if a call came in at 7 p.m. from an established patient who needed an E/M service immediately, you would use the code appropriate for the service and also the code to indicate that the service was provided after office hours:

99212 *Office or other outpatient visit for the evaluation and management of an established patient, which requires at least two of these three key components:*

- *a problem-focused history;*
- *a problem-focused examination;*
- *straightforward medical decision-making.*

Counseling and/or coordination of care with other providers or agencies are provided consistent with the nature of the problem(s) and the patient's and/or family's needs.

Usually the presenting problem(s) are self limited or minor. Physicians typically spend 10 minutes face-to-face with the patient and/or family.

99050 *Services requested after office hours in addition to basic service*

Another example of the use of an adjunct code is for a visit to the emergency room after office hours. Let's say your physician receives a call at 11 p.m. from an established patient suffering acute abdominal distress. Your physician asks the patient to meet him in the emergency room, where he takes an expanded problem-focused history and performs an expanded problem-focused exam. During the exam, he palpates the patient's abdomen and finds no significant pain. Concluding that the patient's distress has been caused by indigestion, he prescribes an over-the-counter antacid and sends the patient home, advising her to call him if the discomfort persists.

This scenario would call for use of the following codes:

99282 *Emergency department visit for the evaluation and management of a patient, which requires these three key components:*

- *an expanded problem-focused history;*
- *an expanded problem-focused examination; and*
- *medical decision-making of low complexity.*

Counseling and/or coordination of care with other providers or agencies are provided consistent with the nature of the problem(s) and the patient's and/or family's needs.

Usually, the presenting problem(s) are of low to moderate severity.

99052 *Services requested between 10:00 PM and 8:00 AM in addition to the basic service*

If the patient in the above example called your physician on **Sunday** at 11 p.m. and he performed the service described, it could be coded in the following way:

99283 *Emergency department visit for the evaluation and management of a patient, which requires these three key components:*

- *an expanded problem-focused history;*
- *an expanded problem-focused examination; and*
- *medical decision-making of moderate complexity.*

Counseling and/or coordination of care with other providers or agencies are provided consistent with the nature of the problem(s) and the patient's and/or family's needs.

Usually, the presenting problem(s) are of moderate severity.

99052	*Services requested between 10:00 PM and 8:00 AM in a d - dition to the basic service*
99054	*Services requested on Sundays and holidays in addition to the basic service*

Your physician may provide a service because the patient has made a special request. For example, the patient asks your physician to see her elderly parent in the parent's home, because the parent is unable to get to the office. The service might be coded as follows:

99347 *Home visit for the evaluation and management of an established patient, which requires at least two of these three key components:*

- *a problem-focused interval history;.*
- *a problem-focused examination; and*
- *medical decision-making that is straightforward or of low complexity.*

Counseling and/or coordination of care with other providers or agencies are provided consistent with the nature of the problem(s) and the patient's and/or family's needs. Usually, the patient is stable, recovering or improving.

99056 *Services provided at the request of a patient in a location other than the physician's office which are normally provided in the office*

Note that the basic service provided in each of the above examples was a history, exam and decision-making process of some type. The adjunct codes are used **in addition to** the visit codes to explain that something about each of the visits was out of the routine (e.g., after regular office hours, on Sunday, at the home of the patient).

Another adjunct code is used specifically for unscheduled office visits. Let's say you receive a call during regular office hours from an established patient who has a foreign body in his eye. Although this condition is not life-threatening, the patient is in acute distress and needs to be seen as soon as possible. You tell him to come in right away, that your physician will "fit him in" (to an already scheduled day). You would code the visit in this way:

*65205** *Removal of foreign body, external eye; conjunctiva superficial*

99058 *Office services provided on an emergency basis*

In this case, you might also consider billing for the use of a surgical tray and an Office/Outpatient visit if appropriate. Review the rules for starred procedures in the Surgery Section. See code 99070, supplies and materials, for non-Medicare patients and HCPCS National Code A4550, surgical tray, for Medicare patients, as well as the pre-op.

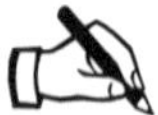

Remember: Each adjunct code has its own distinct price.

CPT's Supply Code: 99070

99070 *Supplies and materials (except spectacles) provided by the physician, over and above those usually included with the supplies or other materials provided*

99070 is the major "supply" code listed in **CPT** (although there are a few supply codes from the Medicine Section under the Ophthalmology subsection). It is a very general code that can be used for supplying anything from an artificial limb to fiberglass for a cast. Because of its generality, using this code to bill for many different kinds of supplies can negatively affect reimbursement.

Code 99071: A Good Public Relations Tool

99071 is a code used to describe books with such titles as ***AIDS, How to Wear Contact Lenses,*** and ***So You're Having a Baby***. These are publications physicians purchase for the education of their patients. The code also includes videotapes, audio cassettes, and pamphlets.

Since most carriers do not pay for supplies associated with the 99071 code, you and your physician will need to decide which of the following approaches to adopt:

a. As with other services you provide, charge patients whose carriers will not pay;

or

b. Include the code on your superbill (if you use one) followed by the "no charge" notation ("N/C"), indicating to your patients that you are giving them something free.

While the former approach appears to be more cost-effective, the latter has considerable value as a public relations tool. It demonstrates to your patients that you are providing something other physicians are not.

Extra Paperwork? Do We Have a Code for You!

99080 *Special reports such as insurance forms, more than the standard reporting form*

This code is to be used when the coder has had to do "extra paperwork," i.e., more than what is done for the average patient. Many people have suggested using this code in cases where a carrier requests extra information in order to process a claim (copies of past charts and histories). If you elect to bill for extra paperwork, however, be sure to inform your carrier beforehand that an additional charge will be assessed for processing such a request.

Submitting your charge to the carrier before you send out the additional information will delay the processing of the major (and probably more expensive) claim you have already submitted. Also keep in mind that you should not withhold information deliberately so that the carrier will write back and request more information. If you have supplied a sufficient amount of information in the first place but additional reports are required (e.g., operative reports or a special report from your physician), you can elect to charge for these reports by using the 99080 code.

Have Code, Will Travel

99082 Unusual travel (e.g., transportation and escort of patient)

Use of this code is warranted when your physician travels a great distance with the patient to a hospital (or elsewhere). Many physicians are now having their patients transported to and from the office or clinic by limousine; this is not an appropriate use of the 99082 code.

You will also recall from our discussion in the Evaluation and Management Section that there are codes there that have to do with patient transport of pediatric patients under the age of 24 months (see codes 99289 and 99290). If you are using these Critical Care Transport codes for the pediatric patients you *do not* also need to add this code, 99082, for unusual travel.

Analysis Adjunct Code

99090 Analysis of clinical data stored in computers (e.g., ECGs, blood pressures, hematologic data)

This code is used when your physician is needed to analyze information generated by a computer. Some computers are available now that will read an entire diagnostic procedure (ECG) and render an interpretation for the physician. When the physician renders an opinion on that interpretation, the opinion is coded with 99090. If there is a more specific **CPT** code available (e.g., a more specific code for cardiographic services, etc.), use it.

STORED AND COLLECTED DATA

Consider the following code that was added to **CPT** for the 2002 book.

99091 *Collection and interpretation of physiologic data (e.g., ECG, blood pressure, glucose monitoring) digitally stored and/or transmitted by the patient and/or caregiver to the physician or other qualified health care professional, requiring a minimum of 30 minutes of time*

Two things should be apparent by looking at this code. The first is that the code includes the "collection" of the data. The second is that it includes the time it took the physician to interpret the data. This is different than the other codes we have seen within the Special Services and Reports subsection of the **CPT** book.

Make sure that when you use each of these, you read the code in full before utilizing it.

QUALIFYING CIRCUMSTANCES FOR ANESTHESIA

As you can see, there are four circumstances that the coder can use to explain the condition of the patient when the anesthesiologist administers the anesthesia.

Let's consider the following example. Suppose you are providing some anesthesia for an 11-month old child who is receiving surgery on his eyes for lazy eye. Your physician would employ the following code in addition to the code for the anesthesia itself.

> *99100* *Anesthesia for patient of extreme age, under one year and over seventy (List separately in addition to the code for primary anesthesia procedure)*

Use of this number will notify the insurance carrier that a special condition applied to this situation.

If you are following along in your **CPT** book in this Special Services and Reports subsection, you will see that immediately after the code 99100 for the Qualifying Circumstances for Anesthesia is a notation that suggests that if you are performing procedures on infants less than one year at the time of surgery, you should check codes 00833, 00834. Unfortunately, when you look up these codes in the Anesthesia section, the code 00833 does not exist.

You will also find codes here in the Medicine Section that are used when the patient receives sedation with or without analgesia.

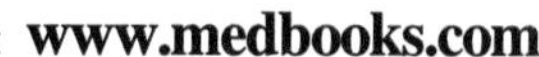

Although there are only a few codes here, many coders miss these numbers because they are not found in the Anesthesia Section.

Home Health Procedures/Services

This subsection was added to the **CPT** for the 2002 book. The codes found here are to be used by the non-physician when he or she sees a patient in the patient's home. "Home" is defined here in **CPT** to mean the patient's residence whether or not that means in an assisted living environment, group home, school, etc. As you may recall, there are home visit codes found in the Evaluation and Management Section in **CPT**. Those codes in the Evaluation and Management Section should be used by physicians to report their services provided to patients in their homes, while the codes found in the Medicine Section can be used by other health care professionals to report the services they do.

For example, let's say that a patient of yours is at home trying to maintain and control her pre-term labor. This mom is on a monitor and must send the monitoring in to a nurse (via the phone) to determine the effectiveness of the drugs being used. If the drugs are not working too well or if she is having trouble with the device used to monitor her contractions, the nurse may decide to use the code 99500 which explains that a home visit was provided to monitor the patient prenatally and to assess fetal heart tones, non-stress tests, uterine monitoring, etc. Codes found in this subsection of Medicine more closely reflect the services being provided than the codes found in the Evaluation and Management Section.

Finally, keep in mind that the codes found here have their own pay scale that is unique to the professionals that provide these services. That is, each of the numbers 99500 through 99600 have their own unique payments which are based not only on the services provided but also on the individuals providing them.

Home Infusion Procedures

This subsection of codes from 99551 through 99600 was added to the 2002 version of **CPT** and significantly changed in the 2003 **CPT** book. Codes found in this subsection can range from home infusion for pain management (99551) through home infusion of additional therapies given on the same day (99569) as well as an unlisted procedure code for this subsection (see 99600). These codes are to be used by a health care professional, and they include a home visit provided by the professional in a single 24-hour time frame. The necessary equipment, solutions, supplies *and* the drugs required to provide the therapy on a 24-hour basis are not included in the descriptions of the codes and should be reported separately. Many, if not all of the codes you will need for the supplies can be found in the **HCPCS Level II National Coding Manual** that was discussed in Chapter Two. If you are providing therapy for the next day, the code can be used a second time.

CPT is very careful to tell the user in the notes found under Home Health Procedures/Services that if you need to apply more than one code from this subsection, you can pick the most complex of the therapies, code for that number and then use the code 99600 for the additional therapies. (The 99600 is a code for unlisted home visit service or procedure.) It is my belief that this is a typo in the 2003 version of the **CPT** book and that what the **CPT** book meant to say was to use the code 99569 for each additional therapy. Here is an example.

Let's say that you provided some infusion for nutrition and in addition to that you also needed to provide some infusion for an antibiotic to eradicate a mild infection that the patient had. You would code in the following way.

99562	*Home infusion for total parenteral nutrition, per visit*
99569	*Home infusion, each additional therapy given on same day (List separately in addition to code for the primary visit) per visit*
J----	*(You would need to pick a code for whatever antibiotic was given to the patient)*

The reason why you would list the more complex code first, followed by the code 99569, is consistent with sound coding practices when you realize that it is not as important to an insurance company computer what happened first, second or third as it is to report the primary services first followed by the secondary or lesser services. Additionally, one can surmise that the plan of the AMA was to provide a mechanism for the insurance carrier to understand the distinction between the 24-hour treatment concept of the first service as is implied by the notes at the beginning of the Home Health Procedures/Services subsection versus other home infusion services provided at the same time.

Summary

CHAPTER TEN

- ✓ The Medicine Section is the last major section of **CPT**.

- ✓ All codes in the Medicine Section begin with the number 9.

- ✓ The services found in the Medicine Section are generally noninvasive where no cutting on anybody happens or where nothing is withdrawn or taken from the patient.

- ✓ If significant separately identifiable Evaluation and Management services are performed at the time an immunization injection is given, an appropriate E/M code may be used in addition to the injection code.

- ✓ When coding for administration of Immune Globulins, Vaccines and Toxoids (codes 90281- 90749), use the immunization administration codes (90471- 90472) in addition to the codes for Immune Globulins, Vaccines, and Toxoids.

- ✓ It is helpful to use the most specific codes for different injectables and supplies.

✓ The Special Services and Reports subsection of the Medicine Section consists of codes 99000 through 99091.

✓ Codes 99000 through 99091, found in the Special Services and Reports subsection, are adjunct codes. That is, they are used only *in addition to* codes for basic services.

✓ Remember to always read the description of the code in its entirety. Failure to read the entire description could result in a failure to correctly identify the procedure and may result in an incorrect payment for the service(s) rendered.

CHAPTER ELEVEN

MODIFIERS

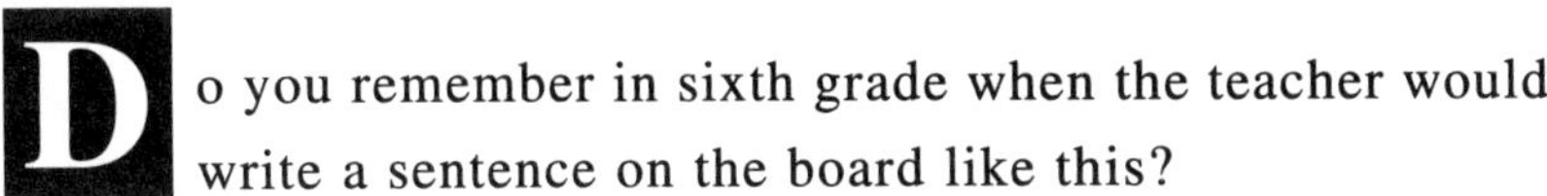

Do you remember in sixth grade when the teacher would write a sentence on the board like this?

Sally has Gucci shoes.

Then she would ask you to name the adjective and the noun?

If your school was like most, you probably learned that an adjective was a word that described or limited a noun or pronoun. That is, in the sentence above, the word Gucci (adjective) describes the kind of shoes (noun) that Sally has.

Another example of an adjective would be the word ***thin***. For example:

Sally is a thin girl.

An adjective gives the reader or listener more of an idea about the noun you are trying to describe than just the use of the noun by itself. For example, you get a different image of Sally if I say, 'Sally is a pretty girl," than if I say 'Sally is a smart girl" or 'Sally is a rude girl," etc.

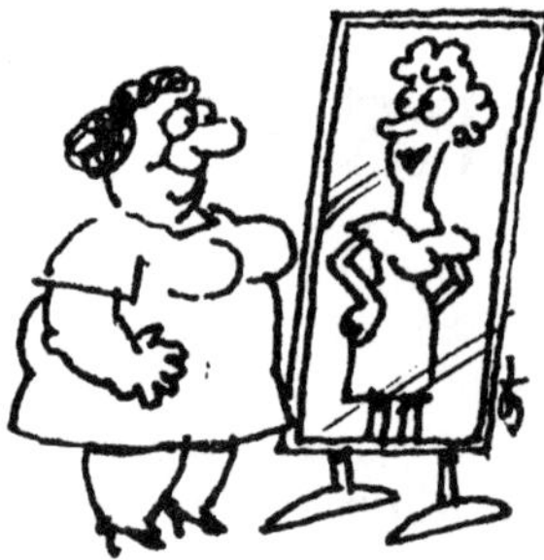

Modifiers should be used accurately. Trying to look on the rosy side will distort the facts and will cause you trouble.

CPT has its own system of adjectives. These are called modifiers. For example:

This is an unusual service.

The adjective here is the word "unusual." The modifier for the word "unusual" is modifier -22. That is, to the computer, the -22 means an unusual service or procedure and is the "adjective" that the computer would understand.

Consider another example:

This is a bilateral procedure.

If you were to underline the adjective and the noun, they would probably be underlined as follows:

This is a bilateral procedure.
adjective noun

In **CPT**, the adjective or modifier for bilateral services is modifier -50.

CPT modifiers are listed in Appendix A. All of these can be useful to you if you know how to use them to better describe the procedures performed by the physician(s).

Learning to use modifiers in **CPT** is like learning to use adjectives in any other language. You must first learn and understand what the adjectives are, and then you must learn how to use them.

Let's suppose you are learning to speak Spanish. In studying this language, you would learn that the placement of the adjective and noun in relation to each other is different from what we find in English.

Consider the following example.

She is a pretty girl.
adjective noun

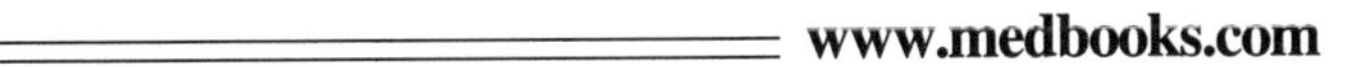

Notice that in English the adjective comes before the noun. In Spanish, however, this sentence reads:

Ella es una <u>muchacha</u> <u>bonita</u>.
noun *adjective*

In the Spanish sentence, the noun comes first (muchacha = girl), and the adjective follows (bonita = pretty).

INDIVIDUAL MODIFIERS

Let's now begin our discussion of individual modifiers. If you will look in your **CPT** book, Appendix A, you will find a complete listing of all of the modifiers that are available to you throughout the book.

TWO WAYS TO WRITE MODIFIERS

As with any language, **CPT** has its own rules. Just remember that in this language, you are learning to communicate with a computer in a way it can understand. Make sure that you are using the correct modifier. For example, it would not be correct to use modifier -52 (Reduced Services) when you really should be using modifier -22 (Unusual Services). As with anything, the better command you have of the language the better the communicator you become.

The following examples make use of a fictitious **CPT** code.

The first way to use a ***CPT*** *code with a modifier is to list the five-digit code and then to list the two-digit modifier.*

2 3 3 3 3 - 2 2

(eight characters)

The second way to write a ***CPT*** *code with a modifier is to list the five-digit code and then list the two-digit modifier without the use of the dash in between the code and the modifier.*

2333322

(seven characters)

Although not using a dash is not stated as an accepted practice by the **CPT** book, many coders employ this method in their coding with great success. Notice that you have only used seven characters here.

2 3 3 3 3 2 2
1 2 3 4 5 6 7

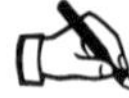

Remember: An adjective, in order to make sense, must refer back to the noun. If we were to say "pretty" without saying what was pretty, it would not make sense to the person with whom we were speaking. Referring back to the procedure, therefore, is important to the modifier. A modifier by itself makes no sense unless it refers back to the procedure that it is supposed to be describing or limiting.

When Using Two or More Modifiers

In the case where two or more modifiers are needed, **CPT** has supplied you with the -99, Multiple Modifiers which can be appended to the procedural code and opens up the insurance company's computer program so that it can read additional modifiers.

Consider the use of a fictitious **CPT** code with the addition of two modifiers:

23333 -99 80-22

Notice that I have only used one line to describe the procedure and its associated modifiers. On the same line, following the modifier -99, I have listed the other two applicable modifiers for this particular case.

Modifier -21: Prolonged Evaluation and Management Services

The use of this modifier applies only to the codes found in the Evaluation and Management Section of **CPT**. As you know from our discussion of the codes found in this section, the great majority of these list some time factor as the average length of the face-to-face encounter. Although time is not considered a "key component" for the selection of an Evaluation and Management code, it does become the controlling factor when the amount of counseling and/or the coordination of care ***exceeds more than 50% of the time*** that it took to perform the history and exam and make the medical decision regarding the patient's diagnosis and/or treatment. If the time spent in counseling and/or coordination of care takes even longer than that listed in the description of the highest level code available for the type of service provided, you would append this modifier to the end of the Evaluation and Management code to show that the encounter took longer than could be normally indicated.

An example may be a comprehensive history and exam performed on a new mute patient who requires an interpreter. If the patient had lots of questions, and the time frame for the exam exceeds the 60-minutes typically provided in this Evaluation and Management Office/Outpatient service for a new patient (which is the highest level for a new patient), then the modifier -21 would be added to the code 99025.

MODIFIER -22: UNUSUAL PROCEDURAL SERVICES

When the service is greater than that described in **CPT**, you can use modifier -22 to help explain to the computer that the service was different from what is usually included in the description of the code.

An example is the woman who had a two hundred-pound ovarian cyst removed. This was an unusual service. That is, there is no code in **CPT** to describe the removal of a cyst of that magnitude. Because of this, the coder can use modifier -22 to describe the unusual aspect of this procedure and to alert the carrier to review that claim by hand.

Due to the modifier -60 (Altered Surgical Field), the modifier -22 is not to be used when the service is "unusual" because of an altered surgical field or formation of adhesions or alteration(s) of normal landmarks on the body due to prior surgery or surgeries, infection or very low weight in infants (under 10 kg) or trauma.

When you submit a modifier -22, Unusual Service, it is important to also submit a special report. A special report describes the unusual circumstances surrounding the procedure and also allows you to present further details of the procedure that will help the carrier determine the payment/reimbursement to be made on the claim.

CPT lists some guidelines on special reports. These instructions can be found in the guidelines of most sections of **CPT**.

Some codes believe it is sufficient to submit an operative report with the claim as a substitute for the special report. This may only be partly true.

Special reports should include:

- Adequate definition or description of the procedure
- Time, effort, and equipment needed to perform the procedure
- Complexity of symptoms
- Final diagnosis
- Pertinent physical findings
- Diagnostic and therapeutic services (including major surgical procedures provided)
- Concurrent (related or unrelated) problems
- Follow-up care

Many claims processors have no medical background. Therefore, it is important to phrase your report in terms that can be understood by the average lay-person. The easier it is for the claims processor to understand your claim and to see justification for paying more for the service, the easier time you will have in getting your reimbursement.

If you have ever paid with a check at a grocery store, you know that the supervisor must approve your check before it is accepted as payment for the goods you just purchased. The use of the modifier -22 is similar in that once it is placed on a claim, that claim cannot be processed until the supervisor has examined it and approved payment. Because the supervisor must check the claim form with the submission of the modifier -22, it is a good idea to use the modifier -22 only when you want the supervisor to manually read your claim form for special cases.

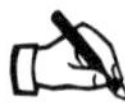

Remember, *you are trying to communicate with someone at the carrier's office who, in all probability, is not a physician.*

Use of the modifier -22 on every claim submitted is similar to the boy who cried wolf. After a while, when the carriers see all of your claims with the -22, they will ignore them. And when, at some point, you have a genuine need for using the modifier -22, that claim will be ignored, too.

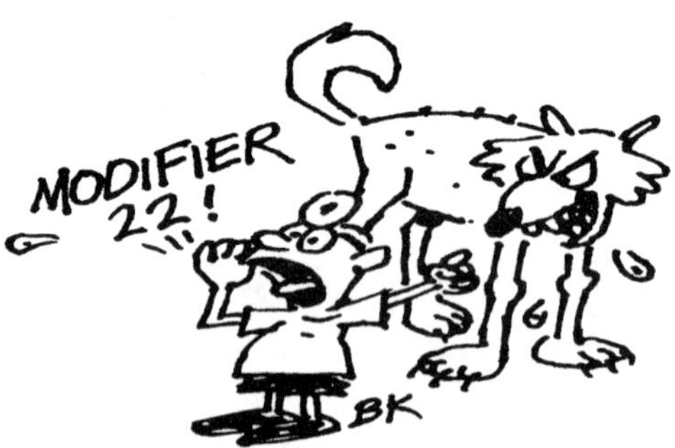

Overuse of the -22 is kind of like the boy who cried wolf...

Modifier -23: Unusual Anesthesia

This modifier is to be used for procedures and services that *normally* require no anesthesia or only local anesthesia but that in this particular case, did require the use of anesthesia. By adding the modifier -23 to the procedure code number, the coder communicates the fact that general anesthesia was provided to the patient.

Modifier -24: Unrelated Evaluation and Management Service by the Same Physician During a Postoperative Period

Modifier -24 addresses Evaluation and Management services that are given to the patient during the follow-up period and are unrelated to the Surgical Package.

As you remember, each of the surgeries listed, with the exception of those that have a star (✱), come complete with their own "package deals." That is, the procedures without a star are similar to "blue plate specials" and include the local infiltration, metacarpal/metatarsal, digital block or topical anesthesia, the Evaluation and Management service that happens immediately prior to and no more than one day before the surgery, the surgery itself, and the normal uncomplicated follow-up care. In other words, everything is included in one price.

Medicare has modified the Surgical Package a bit and included the pre-op (any history and exam done 24 hours prior to the surgery), the surgery, and the postoperative care (that doesn't require a revisit to the operating room) in its Surgical Package for the one price.

For example, let's say that your physician was a family practitioner and a patient came in and had her total obstetrical care (9 months and delivery) at your office. Three days following the birth of her baby, she presents herself to your doctor because she has a lesion on her wrist that has been bothering her. Your physician performs the appropriate history and exam and decides that it (the lesion) is only a common wart and advises this patient to wait another month or so before having the wart removed. This visit obviously had nothing to do with the postoperative follow-up connected with the birth of this woman's baby. It is, therefore, a separate, billable service and would be appropriately billed using the Evaluation and Management code describing the procedure with the addition of the modifier -24 to the end of it.

Modifier -25: Significant, Separately Identifiable Evaluation and Management Service by the Same Physician on Same Day of Procedure or Other Service

The use of the modifier -25 is indicated when a physician has performed a procedure (e.g., a repair of a broken arm) and on the same day, also performed a separate Evaluation and Management service that was warranted based on the patient's problem or condition but that was unrelated to the procedure itself (e.g., examination of a knee lesion). When the Evaluation and Management service is independent and not related to the service or procedure, or when it is above and beyond the usual pre-op or post-op provided, it may be coded in addition to the initial procedure by adding the modifier -25 to the Evaluation and Management code to indicate that the procedure was distinct and connected *or not* connected to the other service.

Modifier -25 may be used with starred *and* global codes. An example would be codes for an office visit that became the "pre-op" for removing a foreign body from the eye (65205* and a starred service). The modifier -25 would be appended to the E/M service.

Another example might be when a physician performs a regular office visit on a child and, during the visit, the mother tells the doctor that the child doesn't seem to hear properly. If the physician proceeds to perform a screening test on the child (92551), the physician would then code the office visit with the modifier -25 attached to the code for the office visit. Note—the diagnosis of the service and the diagnosis of the E/M code may *or may not* be related when using the modifier -25.

MODIFIER -26: PROFESSIONAL COMPONENT

Some procedures listed in **CPT** describe services that were provided by both a physician and a technician. Examples of this may include an x-ray of the humerus, an echocardiography, or a lab procedure.

Suppose a person came into your office and needed an x-ray of the femur. Your physician may request that the technician take the films, but your physician would read them. In other words, the service would have both a professional (physician) component and technical one, and both components would be reported using the same procedure code number.

In some instances, the same office does not perform the two components. The x-rays may be sent to your office so that your physician can interpret them, even though they were not taken at your facility. In cases such as this, addition of the modifier -26 will alert the computer that both service components were not provided by your physician, only the professional component was. Following is an example of how this type of claim should be reported:

73550-26 Radiologic exam, femur, two views

As you can see, with the addition of the modifier -26, the carrier's computer understands that the service for which you are billing was, in fact, that component of the service your physician performed (the reading or interpretation).

Modifier -32: Mandated Service

This modifier applies to services that are "mandated" or "required" by a PRO or third party pay or other appropriate source. For example, let's say that an insurance company will only pay for a certain surgery if the patient gets a second opinion first. The patient comes to your doctor, who renders the second opinion that surgery is warranted. You would take the confirmatory consultation codes and place the modifier -32 at the end of the code to show that the opinion was "required" by the third-party payer.

MODIFIER -47: ANESTHESIA BY SURGEON

The use of this modifier is pretty straightforward; anesthesia (excluding local anesthesia) procedures performed by the surgeon are to be noted by adding the modifier -47 to the procedure code number.

In general, the use of this modifier is very limited. Sometimes, however, a surgeon will provide a type of anesthesia other than local (e.g., regional or general) and will need to report this. By adding the modifier -47 to the end of the procedure for which the anesthesia was needed, the coder is telling the computer that the surgeon (rather than the anesthesiologist) provided the anesthesia.

It is important to note that some carriers want the physician to report the procedure code twice: First the procedure itself and then the fact that the surgeon provided the anesthesia (either general or regional) for the procedure. Check with your major carriers to find out what their policies are regarding the use of this modifier, should you need to employ it.

Modifier -50: Bilateral Procedure

There are times when the physician needs to report services that are performed bilaterally, i.e., performed on both sides of the body. An example is a bilateral breast reconstruction. In this case, **CPT** explains that the appropriate five-digit code describing the first procedure should be listed first.

The second, or bilateral, side should then be reported with the addition of the -50 to the second five-digit procedure code.

For example:

19366 Breast reconstruction with other technique (right side)

19366-50 Breast reconstruction with other technique (left side)

In the 2003 version of **CPT**, there was no longer any indication of whether or not the modifier should be added to the second (bilateral) side. No mention of the addition to the second side was made (as it had been in prior years) nor was there any mention to just add the -50 to the one side only to indicate bilaterality. It is our opinion that you have several choices here. The first is to check with your carrier(s) about what they want, the second is only use the modifiers -RT and -LT on the same code and discussed later in this chapter to indicate right and left sides. The third is to add the modifier -50 as indicated here in

CP"Teach" and finally, you could try adding -50 to the one procedure code to (hopefully) indicate that the separate service was performed bilaterally.

For ophthalmology codes and "ear" codes in the Medicine Section, *bilaterally is assumed* (i.e., it is assumed that when you examine one eye, you will also examine the other). Therefore, use of the bilateral -50 modifier is not required.

MODIFIER -51: MULTIPLE PROCEDURES

The use of this modifier is important when the physician performs more than one surgery at the same operative session or when more than one procedure is provided at the same encounter. For example, the doctor may repair a broken arm and a broken leg at the same time.

When multiple procedures are performed at the same session, **CPT** explains that the major procedure should be reported first and listed by its five-digit **CPT** code. The secondary, additional, or lesser procedures may be reported by listing the procedure code and modifier -51 for each of the additional services.

For example, let's suppose that your doctor provided an intermediate repair on a patient's hands of 7.5 cm, a simple repair of 12.6 cm of the patient's scalp and a complex repair on the patient's trunk of 2.6 cm. The correct codes would be 12032 for the intermediate repair of the hand, 12005 for the 12.6 cm repair of the scalp, and 13101 for the complex repair of the 2.6 cm wound on the trunk.

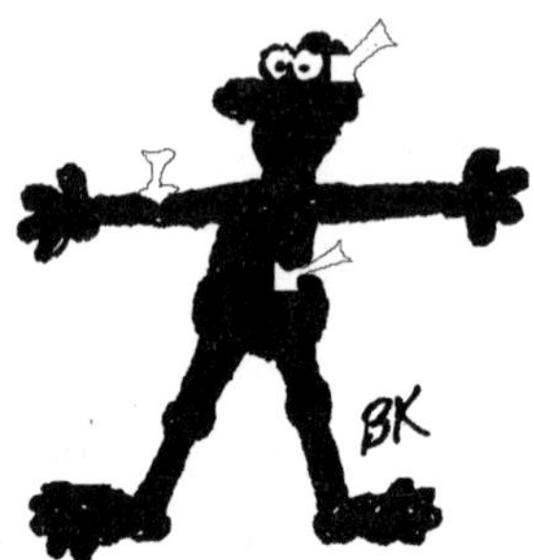

Be careful in coding multiple procedures.

According to **CPT**, you would need to report the major service first. Since the complex repair is the most involved, it would be the major service. Next on the list would be the intermediate repair, and finally the simple repair. On the claim form, you would place the codes and modifiers in the following order.

13101 Complex repair of trunk, 2.6 cm

12032-51 Intermediate repair of hand, 7.5 cm

12005-51 Simple repair of scalp, 12.6 cm

Notice the modifier -51 goes at the end of all secondary procedures and that the major procedure is reported without the addition of the modifier-51.

CPT goes on to state that you do not need to use the modifier -51 on add-on codes (called "sequence codes" by some). These add-on codes may have words like "each additional" as part of the description of its code or the procedures may take into account the same kinds of services on multiple similar body parts.

Consider the following example: Suppose your doctor performed a posterior arthrodesis on a patient's lumbar spine and did two segments in total. Your coding would look like the following:

22612 *Arthrodesis, posterior or posterolateral technique, single level; lumbar(with or without lateral transverse technique)*

✚*22614* *each additional vertebral segment (List separately in addition to the code for the primary procedure)*

Another example might be the following: Say your physician performed an osteotomy on the big toe and on the second one. Your coding would look like this:

64831 *Suture of digital nerve, hand or foot; one nerve*

✚*64832* *each additional digital nerve (List separately in addition to code for primary procedure)*

Because the second toe is "added" on to the service done on the first (same service done on more than one toe), the **CPT** book does ***not*** require you to add the modifier -51 to the secondary code.

It is important for you to look at the codes you are submitting-read their descriptions carefully and think about whether or not the procedures are intimately related (e.g., same procedure-different toe or vertebra). If they are related, the -51 (Multiple Procedures) will not be necessary. If they are not related, you will add the -51 to all additional, secondary or lesser services.

MODIFIER -52: REDUCED SERVICES

Whereas the modifier -22 (Unusual Services) is used to denote circumstances that are abnormally difficult or time-consuming to perform, the -52 (Reduced Services) modifier is used to signify the opposite, that a service was reduced or eliminated in part.

An example of the -52 (Reduced Services) modifier is for an eye or ear exam. Let's suppose that the doctor performed an exam on a patient who only had one eye. The code for the eye exam (e.g., 92002) would be written with the -52 modifier to indicate that the service was partially reduced (i.e., that both eyes were not examined). In addition, a code for examination of the ocular contents would also be used.

Many carriers, physicians, and coders use the -52 (Reduced Service) modifier to indicate reduced fee. ***This is not the correct use*** of the -52 modifier. As you can see by reading the **CPT** book, the -52 modifier clearly indicates reduced services.

Do not confuse the -52 (Reduced Services) modifier with the -53, (Discontinued Procedure) modifier which will be discussed next. The reduced service modifier does not indicate "termination" of a procedure but rather the "reduction" or "elimination" of part of a larger, more global service.

Modifier -53: Discontinued Procedure

Consider, for example, the physician who begins a procedure on a patient. In the middle of the procedure, the patient suffers a myocardial infarction, and the procedure has to be aborted while the patient is resuscitated. In this case, it would not be fair to not bill for the entire procedure, nor would it be fair to obtain full payment for the service.

Use of the modifier -53 shows the computer that you were unable to complete the service and that you may come back at another time to try the service.

Note that the modifier -53 (Discontinued Procedure) is different from the modifier -52 (Reduced Service), in that modifier -53 shows "termination" of a surgical or diagnostic service, whereas modifier -52, (Reduced Service) does not indicate "termination" of a service, but rather "reduction" of a part of the total service.

MODIFIER -54: SURGICAL CARE ONLY
MODIFIER -55: POSTOPERATIVE MANAGEMENT ONLY
MODIFIER -56: PREOPERATIVE MANAGEMENT ONLY

If you recall both the AMA's and the carrier's Surgical Packages and the fact that they include the pre-op, surgery and post-op for one low "blue plate special" price, you can understand the three modifiers listed above.

Breaking the Surgical Package apart, you see the following:

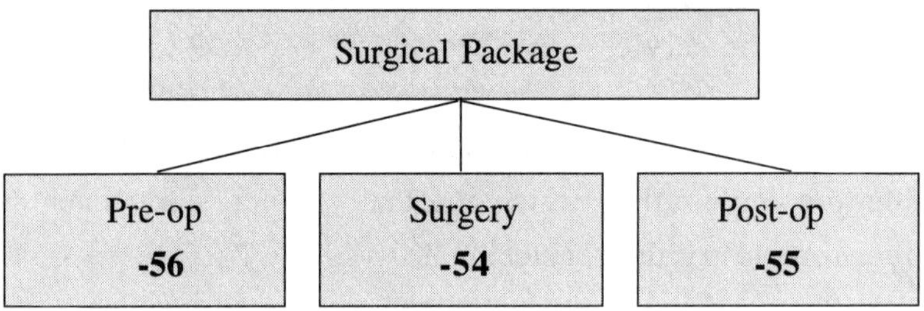

If a physician performed any of the components of the Surgical Package, that particular component could be reported by the addition of the appropriate modifier to the Surgery code.

For example, let's say physician A was going to perform the pre-op and the post-op for a middle ear exploration (see code number 69440) and that physician B was going to perform the surgery only.

The coding would appear as follows:

Physician A (pre-op and post-op)	69440-56
	69440-55
Physician B (surgery only)	69440-54

Now notice that two modifiers are used on the same procedure code number. **CPT** suggests that in a case like this, when two or more modifiers are needed to completely delineate a service, the modifier -99 should be used to signal the computer to open up a new program, enabling it to read the additional modifiers.

MODIFIER -57: DECISION FOR SURGERY

As was discussed in the chapter on Surgery, the Surgical Package (according to most insurance carriers) includes the following:

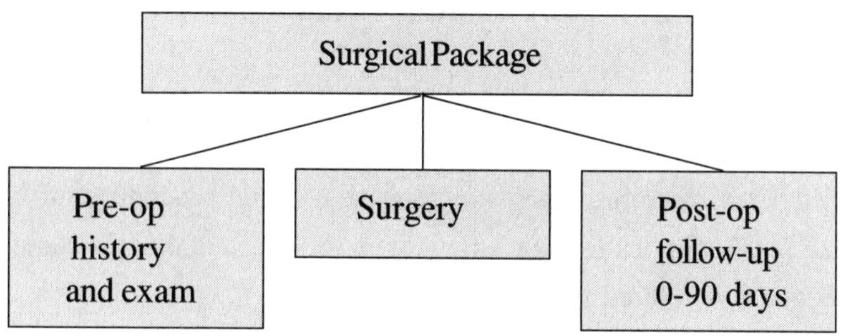

There are some situations, however, in which the patient is evaluated, receives his history and exam and it is decided to do the surgery during that visit .

In cases such as this, modifier -57 can be added to the Evaluation and Management code to show that it was during that particular visit that the physician decided that the surgery should be performed.

An example might be a patient who comes to emergency department following a car accident. The orthopedic surgeon may evaluate the patient and see at this visit that the patient needs to have a fracture of her arm reduced. The Evaluation and Management service could be coded with the addition of the modifier -57 to indicate that this was the visit during which the decision to operate was made. The Evaluation and Management visit would be coded (with the -57) in addition to the code for the fracture repair.

MODIFIER -58: STAGED OR RELATED PROCEDURE OR SERVICE BY THE SAME PHYSICIAN DURING POST-OP PERIOD

This modifier is useful when the coder is trying to show that another procedure may need to be done (will be done) during the post-op time of the first was more extensive than the original procedure or was done for therapy following a diagnostic service, and that the second procedure is related to the first.

For example, let's say that a dog bit your patient and the ripped skin was excised and a tissue expander was placed so that the physician could come back at a later time and perform the reconstructive work. The modifier -58 would be placed on the code(s) used for the reconstructive work to show that they are "related" to the first procedure (in this case, the excision of the skin and the placement of the expander).

Here's another example. Let's say that a patient has come to your office complaining about severe pain in her wrist. You decide that it would be best to perform a diagnostic arthroscopy on her wrist to see if there has been any scarring from a prior surgery she had following an accident a long time ago. You provide the diagnostic arthroscopy and then prescribe that the patient undergo some mild therapy by your physical therapist to make the wrist stronger and hopefully alleviate the pain. You would code the surgery using the code for the diagnostic surgery code (29840) and then you would pick the code for the therapy (e.g., 97110) and add the modifier –58 to the therapy code to indicate that this therapy was related to the diagnostic service.

Modifier -59: Distinct Procedural Service

This modifier is used to report that two (or more) procedures that are not normally done together were done by the same M.D., *on the same day*, at the same or a different session but that they are *unrelated* to each other and are not normally done by the same physician on the same day.

For example, if a diagnostic arthroscopy were performed on the right shoulder (29805) on the same day as an arthroscopy for synovectomy was performed on the left side (29821), you would place the -59 modifier on the end of the 29805 to show that it was not related to the procedure done on the opposite side. Failure to use the modifier could result in a denial of your claim because the computer may think that the smaller service (the diagnostic one, 29805) was part of the larger, 29821 (in this case since they are both arthoscopies).

Remember to place the modifier on the smaller or lesser of the two services.

MODIFIER -62: TWO SURGEONS

Some specific surgical procedures may require the efforts of two surgeons (e.g., an orthopedic surgeon and a neurosurgeon in a Harrington Rod procedure). In this case, both physicians would need to use the same procedure code to describe the procedure.

For example:

22840 *Posterior non-segmental instrumentation (e.g., Harrington rod technique, pedicle fixation across one interspace, atlantoaxial transarticular screw fixation, sublaminar wiring at C1, facet screw fixation)*

Both surgeons would place the modifier -62 after the five-digit code, and both would report the procedure.

Surgeon one:	22840-62
Surgeon two:	22840-62

Use of the modifier -62 is appropriate when each surgeon has a 50% role in the *same procedure.* If two surgeons are working on the same patient but each is working on something different, i.e., one is suturing a lesion and the other is performing a tracheotomy, each physician would report what he or she did without reference to the other doctor (unless the other doctor assisted).

You can use the modifier on as many **CPT** codes as you like as long as both surgeons are working together as primary surgeons and each share an equal role in the procedure.

MODIFIER -63: PROCEDURE PERFORMED ON INFANTS LESS THAN 4 KG

This modifier is similar in concept to the modifier –22 (Unusual Services), in that its use implies that the needs of these small individuals are unique and that some special circumstances are involved (e.g., the complexity of the service is increased as are the risk of complications and physician work). Unlike the modifier –22 which can be used in any of the sections with in the **CPT**, the modifier

–63 should only be used on the surgery codes that begin with 20000 through 69999.

Let's take an example. Suppose you have a newborn patient that is born with a congenital defect of the coronary artery that, without surgery by graft and a cardiopulmonary bypass, will definitely not make it. The surgeon is called in to assess the patient and it is decided that the patient (who only weighs 3.7 kg) should undergo this procedure. Consider how you would code this.

33504-63 Repair of anomalous coronary artery; by graft, with cardiopulmonary bypass-procedure performed on infant less than 4 kg

You will note if you are following along in your **CPT** book and looking at the code 33504 in there, that there are some notations in and around this code that tell you not to use the modifier –63 on the end of the codes 33502, 33503, 33505 and 33506. No reason is given for this request and we were unable to gain any information as to why this would be at the time we went to press. It is noteworthy however, that you should always read the notes in and around the codes you are using to find hints and rules like this that will assist you in filing a clean that will be easily processed.

Modifier -66: Surgical Team

Certain complex surgical procedures require the skills of more than two surgeons. A good example of this is the surgical team required to implant an artificial heart. As with the -62 modifier, the physicians performing the surgery usually have different skills or specialties. Each member of the surgical team would add the -66 modifier to ***all*** of the surgical procedures that he or she performed as part of the team.

Modifier -76: Repeat Procedure by the Same Physician
Modifier -77: Repeat Procedure by Another Physician

One of these two modifiers, depending upon the situation, is to be used when the procedure has been "repeated subsequent to the original service." For example, let's say that your physician reduced a fracture on a child and then, as the child walked out of the room, he fell and the procedure needed to be "repeated." The modifier -76 could be employed. The modifier -77 is similar to the modifier -76,

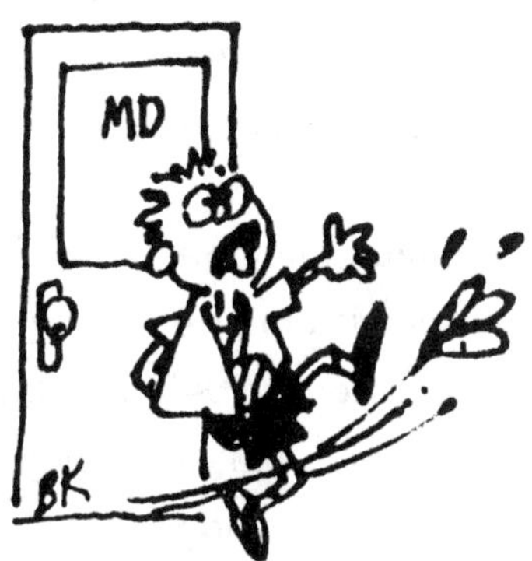

Modifiers -76 and -77 are used when something happens that requires a service to be repeated.

but the modifier -77 indicates that the service repeated was performed by someone other than the physician who provided the initial service.

Modifier -78: Return to the Operating Room for a Related Procedure during the Postoperative Period

The use of the modifier -78 is indicated when the physician for some reason has to go back into the operating room to do another procedure that was related to the first procedure during the period of follow-up (included with the Surgical Package) which has not yet expired. For example, let's say that your physician performs a hysterectomy. Two days following the surgery, the woman begins to hemorrhage, and the patient has to go back to surgery where the laparotomy is reopened. In coding this, you would place the modifier -78 on the end of the code for the laparotomy (i.e., 49002-78).

Another example would be if your physician performed a vitrectomy (mechanical pars plana approach) with endolaser panretinal photocoagulation (67040) and then a month later had to go back to the operating room and complete an epiretinal membrane stripping because of post-op hemorrhage (see 67038). In a case like this, the second procedure (67038) is related to the first and would require the use of the modifier -78.

Modifier –79: Unrelated Procedure or Service by the Same Physician During the Postoperative Period

The use of this modifier is indicated when the procedure that the physician is doing has nothing to do with the other procedure that he or she may have performed. For example, let's say that a physician sets a fracture on day one. Ten days later (still in the postoperative period for the fracture care), the patient returns. This time, however, your physician has to suture a laceration. Notice that the patient falls within the postoperative period for the fracture care, but the laceration repair has nothing to do with the fracture care, and therefore, should be coded and billed separately. Also notice that the service (the laceration repair) is not an Evaluation and Management service. Because of this, you would take the laceration and repair code and add the modifier -79 to the end of it to show that it was unrelated to the postoperative period for the fracture repair.

Note that modifier -79 is conceptually the same as the -24. Both are services that occur during the postoperative period. The differences are that the -24 is an unrelated Evaluation and Management service that occurs during the post op, and the -79 is any other "procedure" that is unrelated and occurs during the post-op.

Modifier -80: Assistant Surgeon
Modifier -81: Minimum Assistant Surgeon
Modifier -82: Assistant Surgeon (when Qualified Resident Surgeon not Available)

These three modifiers are used to describe services rendered by the assistants of the primary surgeon. The modifier -80, (**Assistant Surgeon**), is the most widely used. It is employed by the assistant to the primary surgeon and is placed on the same procedure code that the primary surgeon uses to describe the services he or she provided.

Primary Surgeon:	63688
Assistant Surgeon:	63688-80

The modifier -82 (**Assistant Surgeon [when qualified resident surgeon not available]**), is similar to the modifier -80, but the -82 is to be used in a teaching facility. That is, if no qualified residents are available and the primary surgeon asks a colleague to assist on the surgery, the colleague would use the modifier -82 to indicate that the assistant services were provided in a teaching facility.

The modifier -81 (**Minimum Assistant Surgeon**), can be used in the event of a second assistant. Many coders would like to use the -81 for a nurse employed by the physician who assists in the operation. No official policy regarding this issue has been given by the American Medical Association.

In the book **Medicare RBRVS: A Physician's Guide** (call 1-800-443-7397 or log on to **www.medbooks.com** to obtain), the listing of all the procedures for which Medicare will allow assistants is given in the back of the book.

MODIFIER -90: REFERENCE (OUTSIDE) LABORATORY

The use of this modifier is appropriate when the physician sends work out to a lab (e.g., Pap smears and blood tests). The appendage of the modifier -90 to the end of the procedure/test/smear/specimen that is being tested (e.g., Pap smear) tells the computer that the specimen was not analyzed in the physician's office but was sent to an outside laboratory for processing. However, check with your carrier before using it. Some carriers will not reimburse procedures on which the modifier -90 is appended, as they are expecting to receive the bill from the lab. Still others will not reimburse the physician unless the modifier -90 is added.

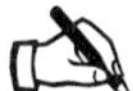

Remember that for all Medicare patients, the lab must do the billing.

MODIFIER -91: REPEAT CLINICAL DIAGNOSTIC LABORATORY TEST

Suppose a patient has undergone major surgery (e.g., total hip replacement or thoracic surgery) and a drainage tube has been placed in the patient to drain excess fluids and blood from the surgical site. The physician may order a hemoglobin to see how the patient is doing. At some point later in the day, the doctor may order another hemoglobin to make sure the patient is still okay. A modifier -91 would be placed on the code(s) for the hemoglobin that was taken subsequent to the first.

MODIFIER -99: MULTIPLE MODIFIERS

Use of the modifier -99 (Multiple Modifiers), has already been discussed under the modifiers -54, -55 and -56. According to **CPT** the modifier -99 is necessary when the coder wants to use more than one modifier. However, most carriers do not require modifier -99. In using the modifier -99, make sure that you place the rest of the modifiers that will follow in order from the highest numeral modifier to the lowest.

An example of the use of the modifier -99 on a bogus **CPT** code follows:

33333 -99 55/54

Anesthesia Physical Status Modifiers

There are six physical status modifiers found in the **CPT** book. These modifiers are used in much the same fashion as we have described the usage of the modifiers above; that is, they are added onto the end of the regular five-digit **CPT** code found in the Anesthesia Section.

An example of how to use these modifiers is the following:

00100-P4

If you also provided services that would warrant the listing of an additional modifier, you would use the physical status modifier first and follow this up with the correct **CPT** nonphysical status modifier. For example, let's say that you provided the anesthesia for an 85 year-old patient who was having a total mastectomy due to cancer. Let's also say that during the procedure the person started to die on the table and so the surgeon stopped the service and discontinued the procedure. As the anesthesiologist, you would code the service in the following way:

0404-99 P4-53 *Anesthesia for procedures on the integumentary system on the extremities, anterior trunk and perineum; radical or modified radical procedures on breast-patient with severe systemic disease that is a constant threat to life-discontinued procedure*

As you can see, as the anesthesiologist you would append the modifier -99 first and then the anesthesia modifier next followed by the other **CPT** modifier(s) as applicable.

Let us describe all six physical status modifiers in detail.

P1 This modifier describes a normal healthy patient and will be used (hopefully) on most of your cases.

P2 This modifier describes a patient that is suffering from a mild systemic disease.

P3 Describes a patient with a severe systemic disease.

P4 Describes a patient with a severe systemic disease that is a constant threat to her life.

P5 This modifier is used to describe a patient who is not expected to survive without the operation.

P6 This modifier describes someone who has been declared "brain dead" and whose organs are being removed for donor purposes.

As you can see, each of these physical status modifiers describe the condition of the patient at the time the anesthesia was administered.

Modifiers Approved For Ambulatory Surgery Center (ASC) Hospital Outpatient Use

There are many modifiers that can be used by both the physician *and* the ambulatory surgical center, (ASC). As we have already discussed the majority of the **CPT** modifiers that apply to the physician, we will list the modifiers that apply to the ASC but only discuss those that are unique to the ASC.

Modifier -25: Significant Separate Identifiable Evaluation and Management Service by the Same Physician on the Same Day as a Procedure or Service

We have already explained the use of this modifier earlier in the chapter.

Modifier -27: Multiple Outpatient Hospital E/M Encounters on the Same Date

Probably the best way to describe this modifier is by giving an example. Let's say that a patient comes into the hospital emergency room and is complaining of stomach pains. The patient appears to be relatively normal and healthy. She is placed back in an examination room of the ER and is examined by the on-call physician there who discovers, after completing a thorough history and exam that the patient is a 35-year old married female (newly wed as of about 8 months) who has been feeling sick for the past 3 weeks on and off.

Today's episode was brought on when she went to work and almost threw up at the morning coffee break time as one of her co-workers was making a new pot of coffee. Since she has not felt well for some time now, one of the co-workers suggested that she be seen (This patient has recently moved to your town and has just recently established her primary care physician but did not call to see if there was any availability at his office.) The ER physician orders some blood work and completes some tests and diagnoses that this patient is pregnant and has been for the past 5 months. During the time it takes for the tests to be completed, she begins to complain of some heavy cramping and vaginal bleeding. The ER doctor administers some turbutaline and calls the on-call OB/GYN who suggests that this patient be moved to the observation unit once she seems stable enough to do so and reports to the ER physician that she will be right in after completing a delivery that she is part of right this second. The patient is moved to the observation unit and the OB/GYN visits her and diagnoses the patient to be in pre-term labor and decides to admit her to the hospital.

As you can see from this example, there are several places (locations) of the hospital that were used for this patient when she was still in an ambulatory or outpatient mode. These included the emergency room and the hospital observation area. In order for the hospital to be able to effectively report the use of these facilities, it can employ the correct codes for the emergency room and the hospital observation area and append the modifier –27 to each of these to indicate that there was more than one hospital E/M encounter that occurred on the same date. The book makes a special point of telling the coder that this modifier is not to be used by the physician to report multiple E/M services on the same date which makes sense when you recall that when a physician provides multiple E/M services on the same date, the smaller services (e.g., office visit) can be grouped with the larger one (e.g., hospital admission) and only the one service that includes the history, exam and medical decision making is reported.

Modifier -50: Bilateral Procedure

The same as described before earlier in this chapter only used by the ASC to denote that two sides of the same service were performed (e.g., bilateral breast reconstructions = 19366 for the right side and 19366-50 for the left as discussed earlier in this chapter.).

Modifier -52: Reduced Services

Again, the same concept as we have described before only in this instance showing that the necessity for the space was reduced because the service was reduced.

Modifier -58: Staged or Related Procedure or Service by the Same Physician During the Postoperative Period

Indicates the usage of the space by the ASC in which a service was planned to be continued at the time of the original service, or that it became more extensive than the original service or that the service described was some sort of therapy for the original service.

Modifier -59: Distinct Procedure Service

Used by the ASC to report that two or more services were done on the same day that may appear to be related but that in reality are distinct and separate services and that the use of the facility was for these purposes.

Modifier -73: Discontinued Out-Patient Hospital/Ambulatory Surgery Center (ASC) Procedure *Prior to* the Administration of Anesthesia

This modifier is unique to the ASC modifiers in that it clearly shows that the procedure had to be aborted before the anesthesia was actually administered. Keep in mind that it would be okay to use this modifier even if the patient had already been sedated...just as long as the patient had not actually received the anesthesia. The use of this modifier on the end of this **CPT** code lets the insurance company know that the work to set up the ASC and prep everything had been done, the patient had been brought in but the full-blown procedure had never been done on the patient due to the discontinuation of the service on the part of the physician. If the patient decides to back out of the service, you would not use this modifier as an insurance company would not pay for this anyway.

Modifier -74: Discontinued Out-Patient Hospital/Ambulatory Surgery Center (ASC) Procedure *After* the Administration of Anesthesia

This modifier is another one of those that is unique to the ASC modifier section and is similar in concept to the one described before (e.g., modifier –73). The difference between these two modifiers is that the –74 modifier lets someone know that the ***anesthesia had already been administered*** when the procedure had been discontinued.

Modifier -76: Repeat Procedure by Same Physician
Modifier -77: Repeat Procedure by Another Physician

Both of these modifiers, when used on a claim for the ASC, will indicate that a service is being repeated subsequent to an original service. The –76 cautions the carrier to look at the fact that the service was already done by the same physician and the –77 cautions the carrier to see that the service being repeated was already done by someone else other than who is performing the service today.

Modifier -78: Return to the Operating Room for a Related Procedure During the Post-Operative Period

As we have already discussed, this modifier is somewhat similar to the repeat procedure modifiers in that we are coming back to do another surgery. The difference here lies in the fact that with the use of this modifier we are wanting to express two things. The first is that the service being done may or may not be the same as the original service and the second is that the patient is returning to the operating room ***during*** the postoperative period. This postoperative period notation is important to the carrier as it indicates that there may have been a complication or that there may be another injury that the patient has sustained that required the return to the operating room.

Modifier -79: Unrelated Procedure or Service by the Same Physician During the Postoperative Period

As you already know from our discussion of the –79 modifier above, the –79 is used to indicate that another procedure or service (e.g., a procedure that has nothing to do with the first service you did) was done during the postoperative time of another service (like a laceration repair done during the postoperative period of a total hip replacement). It is these postoperative time frames and the Global Fee Periods that surround them that get the carriers confused on whether or not they should pay for some services done within the postoperative time frames. Use of the modifiers indicate that the services were legitimate and unrelated to other procedures that have already been done.

Modifier -91: Repeat Clinical Diagnostic Laboratory Test

Used to describe situations in which the test was repeated to make sure that the progress of the patient was proceeding as expected (or not). The modifier -91 is not used when you want to confirm initial results or if you have had problems with the equipment or for any other reason when you just want to re-do the test. There must be a legitimate reason that the test is being re-done and then the use of the modifier is indicated.

Level II (HCPCS/National) Modifiers

There are 31 Level II (or National Code) modifiers that are available in the **CPT** book. Here in **CP"Teach"** we will not take these modifiers in the order in which they appear in the **CPT** book because it will make more sense to you if we keep body parts together (e.g., fingers and toes) as opposed to keeping the modifiers alphabetically.

The Eyes

The modifiers start off with modifiers for the eyes. You will note that these "eye" modifiers start with an "E". There are four eye modifiers; two for the left eye and two for the right, each which is either an upper or lower lid. The modifiers are self-explanatory and you would use them on any procedure that had to do with eyes to describe where the service occurred (i.e., upper or lower lid, left or right eye). Note that it is interesting that upper lids are mentioned with odd numbers (i.e., E1, E3) and lower lids are mentioned with even numbers (i.e., E2, E4) followed in concept with the fact that the left side (i.e., E1, E2) comes before right (i.e., E3, E4).

These modifiers are appended to the end of the procedure code in the same way as regular **CPT** modifiers are added on.

-E1 Upper lid, left

-E2 Lower lid, left

-E3 Upper lid, right

-E4 Lower lid, right

THE FINGERS

The HCPCS modifiers continue with the fingers (hand) and, as you might guess, start off with the letter "F" for fingers. Once again, left hand precedes the right hand for the most part with the exception of the left thumb which is the only modifier for hand that has two alpha characters. The reason for the two alpha-characters is that the modifiers are only two digits. Since there are 10 fingers, you cold not exactly say –F10 as that would make the modifier three digits instead of two.

-F1	Left hand, second digit
-F2	Left hand, third digit
-F3	Left hand, fourth digit
-F4	Left hand, fifth digit
-F5	Right hand, thumb
-F6	Right hand, first digit
-F7	Right hand, second digit
-F8	Right hand, third digit
-F9	Right hand, fourth digit
-FA	Left hand, thumb

The Toes

The third set of Level II modifiers that is pretty easy to understand has to do with the digits of the feet, and, as you might guess, they start off with the letter "T" for toes.

These modifiers do not follow the exact same format as those for the hands but it is similar.

-T1	Left foot, second digit
-T2	Left foot, third digit
-T3	Left foot, fourth digit
-T4	Left foot, fifth digit
-T5	Right foot, great toe
-T6	Right foot, second digit
-T7	Right foot, third digit
-T8	Right foot, fourth digit
-T9	Right foot, fifth digit
-TA	Right foot, great toe

Again, note the two alpha-characters for the description of the right foot, great toe.

Sides of the Body

The next two modifiers talk about on which side of the patient the service took place. That could either be the left or the right side. As might be expected, the left side is modified by using the modifier –LT and the right side is indicated by using the modifier –RT.

-LT left side

-RT right side

The Heart

The next group of modifiers has to do with the heart. These modifiers describe the left circumflex, left anterior descending and right coronary arteries. The left circumflex artery has letters that make sense and is indicated by the two alpha-digits LC for ***l***eft ***c***ircumflex coronary artery. The ***l***eft anterior ***d***escending artery is indicated by the two letters that most closely match its description (the l and the d) hence, modifier –LD. Finally, the modifier for the right coronary artery is –RC as the description implies it should be.

-LC Left circumflex coronary artery (hospitals use with codes 92980-92984, 92995, 92996)

-LD Left anterior descending coronary artery (hospitals use with 92980-92984, 92995, 92996)

-RC Right coronary artery (hospitals use with 92980-92984, 92995, 92996)

AMBULANCES

Finally, we end our discussion of the Level II modifiers with two modifiers that have to do with ambulances. Unlike all the others in this entire group, there is no rhyme or reason to how they chose these. They both start off with the letter “Q” which I suppose you could use to mean “Quick” but what the “M” or the ‘N” could mean is beyond me. You will use them as described below.

-QM Ambulance service provided under arrangement by provider of services

-QN Ambulance service furnished directly by a provider of services

An example of the -QM modifier is the following. Suppose a nursing home were providing the services to a patient and the patient needed an ambulance. The employees of the nursing home, being the “provider”, would call and request an ambulance. The –QN means that the provider of services (in our example, the nursing home) provided the ambulance services themselves.

This concludes our discussion of modifiers. Keep reading them over and over again until you feel comfortable with what each one means and how they can help you further explain to your carrier what happened during each patient encounter.

Summary
CHAPTER ELEVEN

- ✔ Modifiers are adjectives. They further describe or limit the procedure to which they are appended.

- ✔ Modifiers can be written in one of two ways:
    a. Procedure code + dash (-) + modifier: i.e., 19366-20
    b. Procedure code + modifier: i.e., 1936620

- ✔ Check Appendix A in **CPT** for a complete listing of all **CPT** modifiers available to you.

- ✔ Physical Status Modifiers are used to describe the condition of the patient at the time of anesthesia.

- ✔ There are six Physical Status Modifiers. These are appended to the end of the **CPT** code just like the other modifiers.

- ✔ There are many modifiers that apply to both ambulatory surgery centers or hospital outpatient and physician use. There are also some modifiers that are unique to each of these two settings.

✔ The modifiers that are found in the **National Coding Manual** (Level II) are for the most part descriptive of the location in which a procedure or service was provided and often denote the left or right side, the fingers, toes, eyelids or arteries.

CHAPTER TWELVE

Completing Your HCFA 1500 Claim Form for Medicare

Now it's time to take all of the information you have been learning and apply it to the form that most insurance carriers will want you to use. For the physician's office, this form is called the HCFA 1500 claim form. For hospital outpatient coding, this form is called the UB92. The purpose of this chapter will be to explain to you how to correctly fill out the HCFA 1500 form. It will also cover some of the pitfalls that you may encounter if you are working with others who haven't updated their information on the HCFA 1500 claim form.

PURPOSE OF THE HCFA 1500 CLAIM FORM

The HCFA 1500 claim form was created so that Medicare intermediaries (those companies who manage the Medicare program for the federal government in each state) across the country could communicate to each other effectively and so that each carrier would not have to search for the information they needed to correctly process the patient's bill. Before the HCFA 1500 claim form was created, carriers were receiving information about services provided to patients on napkins, handwritten pieces of paper, receipts, superbills and the like, that were not consistent from one physician to another. This caused a delay in the processing of claims as it was difficult for each of the claims, processors to find the **CPT** code(s), the diagnosis code(s), the patient's full name, his Medicare identification number, who provided the services, etc.

In addition to the above, other problems included not being able to read the information that was submitted because it was handwritten. Another issue was receiving a superbill that ended up being the carbon copy of the original and not being able to read that either because the physician may have circled which procedure he/she provided but in doing so, circled two or three of them in one fell swoop! Carriers were literally spending millions of dollars in extra time and personnel due to the significant differences in the many forms that both physicians and patients would submit for payment.

In order to solve these problems, the HCFA 1500 claim form (also known as the Standard Reporting Form) was adopted. This form asked for all of the information that the carriers felt they would need to accurately process the claims.

As you can see by looking at parts of the form on the next few pages, there are 33 general bits of information that need to be filled in. We will take each of these and explain to you how to accurately complete this form.

Please take special care to follow along with this discussion by constantly referring to the HCFA 1500 claim form so that it will make more sense to you. Note that since many of the Medicare carriers also provide insurance plans for non-Medicare patients, they use the HCFA 1500 claim form for both their private and Medicare patients. The HCFA 1500 claim form has also been adopted by the Office of Civilian Health and Medical Program of the Uniformed Services (OCHAMPUS).

COMPLETING THE HCFA 1500 CLAIM FORM

Space 1. As you can see by looking at **Space 1** on the next page, there are several types of insurances that the patient may have. These include (but are not limited to) the following:

a. Medicare
b. Medicaid
c. Champus
d. Champva
e. Group Health Plan

f. FECA Black Lung

g. Other

PLEASE DO NOT STAPLE IN THIS AREA

APPROVED OMB-0938-0008

CARRIER

PICA

HEALTH INSURANCE CLAIM FORM

PICA

1. MEDICARE (Medicare #) / MEDICAID (Medicaid #) / CHAMPUS (Sponsor's SSN) / CHAMPVA (VA File #) / GROUP HEALTH PLAN (SSN or ID) / FECA BLK LUNG (SSN) / OTHER (ID)		1a. INSURED'S I.D. NUMBER (FOR PROGRAM IN ITEM 1)	
2. PATIENT'S NAME (Last Name, First Name, Middle Initial)	3. PATIENT'S BIRTH DATE MM DD YY / SEX M F	4. INSURED'S NAME (Last Name, First Name, Middle Initial)	
5. PATIENT'S ADDRESS (No., Street)	6. PATIENT RELATIONSHIP TO INSURED: Self / Spouse / Child / Other	7. INSURED'S ADDRESS (No., Street)	
CITY / STATE	8. PATIENT STATUS: Single / Married / Other	CITY	STATE
ZIP CODE / TELEPHONE (Include Area Code) ( )	Employed / Full-Time Student / Part-Time Student	ZIP CODE	TELEPHONE (INCLUDE AREA CODE) ( )

FORMATION

It is important for you to check off the appropriate box depending on the kind of insurance that the patient has, and then, depending on the kind, move over to **Space 1a** and fill in the insured's identification number. Note that the number that you fill in for **Space 1a** will depend on what you checked off in **Space 1**. For example, if you checked off CHAMP-VA, you will need to place the patient's VA file number in **Space 1a**. If you checked off Group Health Plan, you will need to make sure that you list the patient's social security number or some other identification number.

If you checked Medicare, make sure that you list the patient's Medicare Health Insurance Claim Number (HICN),whether Medicare is the primary or secondary payer.

Space 2. As explained in the verbage on the form, you are supposed to enter the patient's full name. Remember that the ***full*** name is very important. As many patients have the same name, the use of a middle initial is very helpful to your carrier in identifying patients of the same appellation. Be sure to use the LAST name first, followed by the first name and middle initial.

Space 3. This is the space where you are supposed to enter the patient's birthday. In doing so, make sure that you list the birth date with the month, date, and four-digit year (08/17/1919) as opposed to listing August 17, 1919, for example. Also make sure that you ***list all eight digits of the patient's birthday***. Using less than eight digits may confuse the carrier and cause a delay in the processing of your claim.

It is also important that you check off the appropriate box denoting the sex of the patient. Failure to do this could also result in a slowed or unprocessed claim.

Space 4. If there is an insurance that is the primary insurance (and takes precedence over Medicare), either through the patient herself or the patient's spouse, make sure that you complete this space. If the patient and the insured are the same, mark the word SAME in the space provided.

If the patient and insured are different (i.e., the patient is not the one who holds the policy), list the name of the insured here. For example, let's say that the patient is a female homemaker named Diane Taceeya and her husband, Ronald Taceeya, is employed at the local factory. Let's also say that being employed there, he has a group health plan that is very good. You would need to make sure that you enter Mr. Taceeya's full name (first name, middle initial, and last name) in **Space 4** so that when this claim is processed, the carrier will know whose policy to verify and pay from. Be sure to use the LAST name first, followed by the first name and middle initial.

At this time, you may want to also complete **Space 6**, which asks for the relationship of the patient and the insured, and **Space 7**, which asks for the insured's address.

Space 5. Here is where you are supposed to give the name and address of the patient. Sometimes this may be different than the insured. That is okay. Make sure to list the name and address of the patient him/ herself. Do not try to crowd all of the information on one line. Note that there are multiple lines for you to complete the address. On the first line, list the street address and the apartment number (if any), and then, on the second line, list the city and state. List the zip code and the patient's 10-digit phone number on the third line.

hint

Failure to complete any of these lines could result in a delay or denial of your claim.

Space 6. This one should be easy. All they are asking for here is the patient's relationship to the insured. If the patient and the insured are divorced, but the patient is still receiving benefits from the ex- spouse, mark the space for "other." It is sometimes helpful to complete this space right after you complete **Space 4**, listing the insured's name.

Space 7. Completing this space requires completion of the insured's address. As was requested in **Space 5**, make sure that you do not try to cram everything on one line. There is plenty of space for you to list all of the information requested. Do not forget to list any apartment number (if there is one) as well as the insured's zip code.

Space 8. Here is where you should place the patient's status, i.e., whether he is married, single, or other (divorced, widowed, or separated). You will also need to check the appropriate box that lists whether the patient is employed, a full-time student, or a part-time student.

Employed ☐ Full-Time Student ☐ Part-Time Student ☐

9. OTHER INSURED'S NAME (Last Name, First Name, Middle Initial)
10. IS PATIENT'S CONDITION RELATED TO:
11. INSURED'S POLICY GROUP OR FECA NUMBER

a. OTHER INSURED'S POLICY OR GROUP NUMBER
a. EMPLOYMENT? (CURRENT OR PREVIOUS) ☐ YES ☐ NO
a. INSURED'S DATE OF BIRTH MM | DD | YY SEX M ☐ F ☐

b. OTHER INSURED'S DATE OF BIRTH MM | DD | YY SEX M ☐ F ☐
b. AUTO ACCIDENT? PLACE (State) ☐ YES ☐ NO
b. EMPLOYER'S NAME OR SCHOOL NAME

c. EMPLOYER'S NAME OR SCHOOL NAME
c. OTHER ACCIDENT? ☐ YES ☐ NO
c. INSURANCE PLAN NAME OR PROGRAM NAME

d. INSURANCE PLAN NAME OR PROGRAM NAME
10d. RESERVED FOR LOCAL USE
d. IS THERE ANOTHER HEALTH BENEFIT PLAN? ☐ YES ☐ NO *If yes*, return to and complete item 9 a-d.

READ BACK OF FORM BEFORE COMPLETING & SIGNING THIS FORM.

12. PATIENT'S OR AUTHORIZED PERSON'S SIGNATURE I authorize the release of any medical or other information necessary to process this claim. I also request payment of government benefits either to myself or to the party who accepts assignment below.

SIGNED ____ DATE ____

13. INSURED'S OR AUTHORIZED PERSON'S SIGNATURE I authorize payment of medical benefits to the undersigned physician or supplier for services described below.

SIGNED ____

PATIENT AND INSURED INFORMATION

14. DATE OF CURRENT: ILLNESS (First symptom) OR
15. IF PATIENT HAS HAD SAME OR SIMILAR ILLNESS
16. DATES PATIENT UNABLE TO WORK IN CURRENT OCCUPATION

Space 9: You will only need to complete any of this space if:

a. You are a participating physician or you are a participating supplier; ***AND***

b. The beneficiary wishes to assign his/her benefits (under a **Medigap policy**) to the participating physician or supplier.

If these conditions do ***not*** apply, skip to **Space 10**.

MEDIGAP: THE SUPPLEMENTAL INSURANCE POLICY

For Medicare, **Space 9** is primarily to find out if there is a person enrolled in a Medigap policy. "Medigap" is a supplemental insurance policy (or other health benefit) offered by a private entity to people entitled to Medicare benefits. It is specifically designed to supplement Medicare benefits (or fill in the "gaps" in Medicare coverage). Medigap provides payment for some of the charges that Medicare does not pay due to:

a. Applicability of deductibles;
b. Co-insurance amounts;
c. Other limitations imposed by Medicare.

Medigap excludes the following:

a. Limited benefit coverage available to Medicare beneficiaries, such as "specified disease" or "hospital indemnity";
b. A policy or plan offered by an employer to employees or former employees;
c. A policy or plan offered by a labor organization to members or former members.

You ***should not*** list other supplemental insurance in this space for Medicare. If the private insurance companies contract with Medicare, Medicare will automatically and electronically send them the information they need to process their portion of the patient's bill. If there is no such contract between the private insurance company and Medicare, the patient will have to submit his or her own supplemental claim.

If the patient has met the conditions listed above and needs for you to complete this portion of the form (**Space 9** and its adjuncts), make sure that you list the patient's last name first, followed by her first, and then her middle initial. There may come a time in the future when this space will be used for supplemental insurance plans.

( )	Student ☐ Student ☐	( )
9. OTHER INSURED'S NAME (Last Name, First Name, Middle Initial)	10. IS PATIENT'S CONDITION RELATED TO:	11. INSURED'S POLICY GROUP OR FECA NUMBER
a. OTHER INSURED'S POLICY OR GROUP NUMBER	a. EMPLOYMENT? (CURRENT OR PREVIOUS) ☐ YES ☐ NO	a. INSURED'S DATE OF BIRTH MM | DD | YY SEX M ☐ F ☐
b. OTHER INSURED'S DATE OF BIRTH MM | DD | YY SEX M ☐ F ☐	b. AUTO ACCIDENT? PLACE (State) ☐ YES ☐ NO	b. EMPLOYER'S NAME OR SCHOOL NAME
c. EMPLOYER'S NAME OR SCHOOL NAME	c. OTHER ACCIDENT? ☐ YES ☐ NO	c. INSURANCE PLAN NAME OR PROGRAM NAME
d. INSURANCE PLAN NAME OR PROGRAM NAME	10d. RESERVED FOR LOCAL USE	d. IS THERE ANOTHER HEALTH BENEFIT PLAN? ☐ YES ☐ NO ***If yes**, return to and complete item 9 a-d.*
READ BACK OF FORM BEFORE COMPLETING & SIGNING THIS FORM. 12. PATIENT'S OR AUTHORIZED PERSON'S SIGNATURE I authorize the release of any medical or other information necessary to process this claim. I also request payment of government benefits either to myself or to the party who accepts assignment below. SIGNED ____	DATE ____	13. INSURED'S OR AUTHORIZED PERSON'S SIGNATURE I authorize payment of medical benefits to the undersigned physician or supplier for services described below. SIGNED ____
14. DATE OF CURRENT: ILLNESS (First symptom) OR	15. IF PATIENT HAS HAD SAME OR SIMILAR ILLNESS.	16. DATES PATIENT UNABLE TO WORK IN CURRENT OCCUPATION

PATIENT AND INSURED INFO

In **Space 9a**, you should list the policy and group number of the Medigap insured. Make sure that when you do this, you place either the abbreviation for Medigap "MG" or "MGAP" or the actual word "Medigap" itself before you put in the number.

In **Space 9b**, as in other spaces, list the person's 8-digit birthday with the month listed first, followed by the date, and, finally, the year. Note that the year will require all four digits (i.e., year 2000 or 2001, etc.). This is the same method that was used in **Space 3**.

You will leave **Space 9c** blank if a Medigap Payer Identification is entered in **Space 9d**. If you do not enter the Medigap Payer Identification number in **Space 9d**, make sure that in **Space 9c** you list the address of the Medigap insurance program. Since the space here is rather small, you would use abbreviations to denote the address and you would list it all in one line. For example, you might write 101 W. Buckingham Rd. TX 75081. (Note that a city is not listed here. Don't worry about that as Medicare knows what the city is based on the state and zip code you listed).

On the HCFA 1500 claim form, **Space 9d** looks like it wants you to fill in the Medigap insurance program or name. THIS IS NOT REALLY WHAT THEY PREFER.

If you have the 9-digit payer identification number of the Medigap insurer, Medicare would prefer that you enter this number in **Space 9d**. If you do not have it, then enter the name of the Medigap insurance program or plan.

hint

If you are a participating supplier or provider, and the beneficiary wants Medicare data forwarded to a Medigap insurer, all information in ***Spaces 9, 9a, 9b, and 9d*** *must be complete and accurate. Otherwise, the Medicare carrier will not forward the claim to the Medigap insurer.*

The next few spaces, **Spaces 10a** through **10c**, requesting information on the patient's condition, are fairly simple to complete. All you have to do is check YES or NO after the questions listed on the form to indicate whether the person received treatment (which will be described in **Space 24** by the **CPT** codes that you choose) due to a car accident, employment, or other accident. Make sure that you identify in the space provided the state in which the problem/ condition occurred, using the abbreviation for the state (e.g., TX). If you do check a YES here in **Space 10**, relating to how the patient's condition developed, there may be another form of insurance that becomes the primary insurance. In other words, let's suppose that a Medicare beneficiary was in an automobile accident caused by a teen who had Allstate insurance. By checking YES under the space provided to indicate that the injury was caused by an auto accident (see **Space 10b**), Medicare would know that they need to look for another insurance company which may take precedence over Medicare. If this is true and there is another "primary" insurance, make sure to indicate that on the HCFA 1500 by completing the box in Space 11.

Space 11. Insured's Policy Group or FECA number. **This space MUST be completed for Medicare.** Completing this space for Medicare shows that the physician or supplier has made a "good faith" effort to find out from the patient if there is another insurance which may take precedence over Medicare (or which may be considered the "primary" insurance company). Obviously, if there is another company that is responsible for the majority of the bill, it stands to reason that Medicare is going to want them to pick up the majority of the tab. If not, Medicare will know that they will be responsible for the majority of the bill.

WHEN MEDICARE IS NOT THE PRIMARY INSURER

If there is an insurance company primary to Medicare, you will need to enter the insured's policy number (or group number) in **Space 11**. Example of types of insurance that may be considered "primary" to Medicare follow:

I. Group Health Plan
   a. Working Aged;
   b. Disability (Large Group Health Plan); and
   c. End Stage Renal Disease;

II. No Fault and/or other Liability;

III. Work Related Illness/Injury
   a. Worker's Compensation;
   b. Black Lung; and
   c. Veterans' Benefits.

The patient may report that he had a primary insurance company (e.g., when he worked at the local plant one month ago) but that he is now retired. If the patient reports an event like this, which may have terminated the primary insurance, mark the word "NONE" in **Space 11**.

If you do find that there is an insurance company that is primary to Medicare, and you decide to send in a HCFA 1500 claim form through the mail (as opposed to sending it via your computer), you will need to make sure that you also send a copy of the explanation of benefits from that primary insurance company to Medicare so that they can properly process this claim.

Although some of the time it seems as if you are duplicating the information that you have already completed somewhere else on the form, remember that it is to your best advantage to do it again in order to be paid. Anytime information is left out, an insurance company can choose to deny your claim. This only results in lost payments for your office or clinic and causes problems for you and your patients. It could also impact the credit histories of your patients due to the fact that you may send them to a collection agency based on unpaid accounts. Remember, you initiated the problem by not completing the form properly.

If there is no insurance primary to Medicare, you may skip to **Space 12** and leave everything in **Space 11** blank.

( )

Employed ☐ Full-Time Student ☐ Part-Time Student ☐

( )

9. OTHER INSURED'S NAME (Last Name, First Name, Middle Initial)

a. OTHER INSURED'S POLICY OR GROUP NUMBER

b. OTHER INSURED'S DATE OF BIRTH MM | DD | YY SEX M ☐ F ☐

c. EMPLOYER'S NAME OR SCHOOL NAME

d. INSURANCE PLAN NAME OR PROGRAM NAME

10. IS PATIENT'S CONDITION RELATED TO:

a. EMPLOYMENT? (CURRENT OR PREVIOUS) ☐ YES ☐ NO

b. AUTO ACCIDENT? ☐ YES ☐ NO PLACE (State)

c. OTHER ACCIDENT? ☐ YES ☐ NO

10d. RESERVED FOR LOCAL USE

11. INSURED'S POLICY GROUP OR FECA NUMBER

a. INSURED'S DATE OF BIRTH MM | DD | YY SEX M ☐ F ☐

b. EMPLOYER'S NAME OR SCHOOL NAME

c. INSURANCE PLAN NAME OR PROGRAM NAME

d. IS THERE ANOTHER HEALTH BENEFIT PLAN? ☐ YES ☐ NO *If yes*, return to and complete item 9 a-d.

READ BACK OF FORM BEFORE COMPLETING & SIGNING THIS FORM.

12. PATIENT'S OR AUTHORIZED PERSON'S SIGNATURE I authorize the release of any medical or other information necessary to process this claim. I also request payment of government benefits either to myself or to the party who accepts assignment below.

SIGNED ________ DATE ________

13. INSURED'S OR AUTHORIZED PERSON'S SIGNATURE I authorize payment of medical benefits to the undersigned physician or supplier for services described below.

SIGNED ________

PATIENT AND INSURED INFOR

14. DATE OF CURRENT: ILLNESS (First symptom) OR

15. IF PATIENT HAS HAD SAME OR SIMILAR ILLNESS.

16. DATES PATIENT UNABLE TO WORK IN CURRENT OCCUPATION

In **Space 11a** for date of birth, once again, make sure that the insured's date of birth is given using all eight digits of the birth date ***if it is different than what is in Space 3***. For example, August 17, 1919 would be written as 08/17/1919. Also, denote in this box the sex of the patient.

Does Retirement Make a Difference?

Space 11b asks for the employer's name or school name. If the patient is employed, enter this information here. However, if the patient is retired, you need to enter in a retirement date, preceded by the word "RETIRED" (e.g., RETIRED 01/01/2000). Make sure all of this information is complete if there is an insurance company primary to Medicare.

In **Space 11c**, the form calls for the insurance plan name or program name. For Medicare patients, it is preferred that you enter in the payer's identification number (for the primary insurance company). If no such number exists, enter in the COMPLETE primary payer's program or plan name. It is important to check the primary payer's claims processing address and make sure that if it isn't already on the explanation of benefits (EOB) (given to you by the patient or received in the mail) that you record this address directly on the EOB.

Space 11d, which asks about other health benefit plans, is not required by Medicare. When using the HCFA 1500 form for non-Medicare patients, enter in the information on whether or not there is another health benefit plan by completing this space.

Space 12. Patient's signature. This space can be completed in a variety of ways. You may have the patient (or authorized representative):

a. Sign and date the form using the six-digit date (MM/DD/YY) or an eight-digit date (MM/DD/YYYY) or even an alphanumeric date (January 1, 2003).

b. Sign a statement that is retained by you (the physician, supplier, or provider). This statement releases the medical information necessary to process the claim(s) and also authorizes payment of the claim to the provider, physician, or supplier when the provider, supplier, or physician "accepts assignment" of the claim (agrees to accept benefits paid on the claim as payment for the claim). Once such a statement has been signed, it will remain in effect until the patient or his of her authorized representative revokes the statement. An original of this statement should be maintained in the patient's file. If you choose to have the patient sign such a statement, you will need to fill in **Space 12** with the words "signature on file".

If the form is signed by an *authorized representative* of the patient, make sure that this person is in compliance with the rules outlined in the **Medicare Carrier's Manual** for such a representative. You can obtain the **Medicare Carrier Manual** by writing or calling the

Government Printing Bookstore (located in every major metropolitan area).

If the form is signed by a patient using an "X" (usually by an illiterate or handicapped patient), there must be a representative there that witnesses the signature. Usually, this would be the person who is responsible for handling the insurance claims forms processing in your office, the office manager, or someone like that.

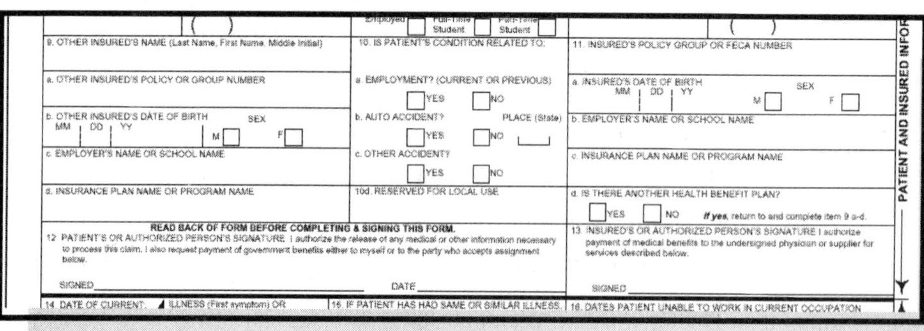

Employed ☐ Full-Time Student ☐ Part-Time Student ☐

9. OTHER INSURED'S NAME (Last Name, First Name, Middle Initial)
a. OTHER INSURED'S POLICY OR GROUP NUMBER
b. OTHER INSURED'S DATE OF BIRTH MM | DD | YY SEX M ☐ F ☐
c. EMPLOYER'S NAME OR SCHOOL NAME
d. INSURANCE PLAN NAME OR PROGRAM NAME

10. IS PATIENT'S CONDITION RELATED TO:
a. EMPLOYMENT? (CURRENT OR PREVIOUS) ☐ YES ☐ NO
b. AUTO ACCIDENT? ☐ YES ☐ NO PLACE (State)
c. OTHER ACCIDENT? ☐ YES ☐ NO
10d. RESERVED FOR LOCAL USE

11. INSURED'S POLICY GROUP OR FECA NUMBER
a. INSURED'S DATE OF BIRTH MM | DD | YY SEX M ☐ F ☐
b. EMPLOYER'S NAME OR SCHOOL NAME
c. INSURANCE PLAN NAME OR PROGRAM NAME
d. IS THERE ANOTHER HEALTH BENEFIT PLAN? ☐ YES ☐ NO ***If yes***, return to and complete item 9 a-d.

READ BACK OF FORM BEFORE COMPLETING & SIGNING THIS FORM.

12. PATIENT'S OR AUTHORIZED PERSON'S SIGNATURE I authorize the release of any medical or other information necessary to process this claim. I also request payment of government benefits either to myself or to the party who accepts assignment below.

SIGNED ________ DATE ________

13. INSURED'S OR AUTHORIZED PERSON'S SIGNATURE I authorize payment of medical benefits to the undersigned physician or supplier for services described below.

SIGNED ________

PATIENT AND INSURED INFOR

14. DATE OF CURRENT: ILLNESS (First symptom) OR
15. IF PATIENT HAS HAD SAME OR SIMILAR ILLNESS.
16. DATES PATIENT UNABLE TO WORK IN CURRENT OCCUPATION

Space 13. Insured or authorized person's signature. Like **Space 12**, this space will need to be signed if there is a Medigap form of insurance. A signature in this space authorizes payment of the Medigap benefits to the physician, supplier, or provider if the appropriate information is listed in **Space 9** and its subdivisions. The same concept as was discussed for **Space 12** applies here. That is, it is okay for you to maintain a statement signed by the patient assigning non-Medicare benefits to the physician, supplier, or provider if it is separate from the one assigning Medicare benefits to the physician, supplier, or provider. The statement and its assignment must be insurer specific. That is, if the patient started off with one Medigap insurer and you had a signed statement from the patient assigning benefits for that insurance company, it could not be transferred to another insurer if the patient switched. The statement may also state the that the authorization of benefits applies to all occasions for service until revoked by the patient or authorized representative.

Let's now move to **Spaces 14 through 23.**

14. DATE OF CURRENT: MM | DD | YY — ILLNESS (First symptom) OR INJURY (Accident) OR PREGNANCY(LMP)
15. IF PATIENT HAS HAD SAME OR SIMILAR ILLNESS. GIVE FIRST DATE MM | DD | YY
16. DATES PATIENT UNABLE TO WORK IN CURRENT OCCUPATION MM | DD | YY FROM — TO MM | DD | YY
17. NAME OF REFERRING PHYSICIAN OR OTHER SOURCE
17a. I.D. NUMBER OF REFERRING PHYSICIAN
18. HOSPITALIZATION DATES RELATED TO CURRENT SERVICES MM | DD | YY FROM — TO MM | DD | YY
19. RESERVED FOR LOCAL USE
20. OUTSIDE LAB? YES NO — $ CHARGES
21. DIAGNOSIS OR NATURE OF ILLNESS OR INJURY. (RELATE ITEMS 1,2,3 OR 4 TO ITEM 24E BY LINE)
1. ___ . __
2. ___ . __
3. ___ . __
4. ___ . __
22. MEDICAID RESUBMISSION CODE — ORIGINAL REF. NO.
23. PRIOR AUTHORIZATION NUMBER
24. A B C D E F G H I J K

Space 14 asks for the date of the current illness (first symptom) or date of injury (accident) or pregnancy (denoted by the date of the last menstrual period). As you have done before on the form, list the six-digit date (MM/DD/YY) or the eight-digit date (MM/DD/YYYY). If you are coding for a chiropractor, enter in the six or eight-digit date of the initiation of the course of treatment.

In **Space 15**, you are asked to indicate whether the patient has had the same or similar illness. This information is not required by

Medicare and, as such, should be left blank if you are filing for a Medicare patient. You will want to complete this information for non-Medicare carriers, if you have it available.

Space 16 talks about the dates the patient was unable to work. It is applicable if the patient is employed and is unable to work due to the problem or condition. As an entry in this spot may indicate "employment-related" coverage (and it may be, therefore, that Medicare will not be the primary insurer), it is important to fill in either the six or eight-digit date (as we have discussed before), indicating the date that the patient is (or was) unable to work.

ORDERING AND REFERRING PHYSICIANS

Space 17. If the patient was ***referred to, or a service ordered by*** your office by another physician, please indicate that physician's name and the National Provider Identifier (NPI). For Medicare purposes, a referring physician is one who requests an item or service for the patient where payment for such service or item may be made under the Medicare program. Likewise, an ordering physician is one who orders *non-physician* services for the patient, such as durable medical equipment, diagnostic services, laboratory tests, or pharmaceutical services.

Back in 1992, the Federal Government ordered that physicians could not refer themselves. In basic layman's terms this meant that a patient had to have the right to get "ordered" services (e.g., glasses, durable medical equipment, etc.) from anyone she chose. Otherwise, the physicians could order things for patients and directly receive the benefit of getting the extra money from the supply of that item. This ordering/referring requirement became effective as part of the Social Security Act in January of 1992.

Ordering/referring requirements extend to cover:

a. parenteral and enteral nutrition;
b. immunosuppressive drug claims;
c. diagnostic lab services;
d. diagnostic radiology services;
e. consultative services;
f. durable medical equipment.

All claims for ordered or referred services, whether included or not in the preceding list, must show the ordering/referring physician's name and National Provider Identifier. An example would be a surgeon who must complete **Space 17** and **17a** (name of referring physician or source) when another physician has referred the patient to him.

When the ordering physician is also the performing physician, as is often the case with in-office clinical lab tests, the performing physician's name and assigned NPI must appear in **Spaces 17** and **17a**.

Obtaining an NPI

A National Provider Number (NPI) is essential for all physicians who order for or refer Medicare beneficiaries, even if they never bill

Medicare directly. If you do not have an NPI, you will need to contact your Medicare carrier directly.

If the ordering or referring physician has not been assigned an NPI, she will need to use one of the surrogate NPI's listed below. Permission to use a surrogate NPI depends on the circumstances of use and is only available for use until the physician is assigned her own NPI. Claims with surrogate NPIs will be tracked and possibly audited by Medicare.

Surrogate NPI's have eight digits. It is important to use all eight digits when reporting an NPI. Surrogate NPIs, for those physicians without one, are as follows:

a. **Residents**: RES00000

b. **Retired physicians** who were not issued an NPI:RET00000

c. **Physicians** serving in the **Department of Veterans Affairs** or **U.S. Armed Services**: VAD00000

d. **Physicians** in the **Public Health** or **Indian Health Services**: PHS00000

e. **Nurse practitioners, clinical nurse specialists, or any non-physician practitioner** in a non-metropolitan statistical area, who is state-licensed to order medical services or refer patients to Medicare providers without the approval or collaboration of a supervising physician: NPP00000

f. **Physicians who have not been assigned an NPI** and who do not meet one of the criteria above: OTH00000 (until an individual NPI is assigned).

14. DATE OF CURRENT: MM | DD | YY — ILLNESS (First symptom) OR INJURY (Accident) OR PREGNANCY(LMP)
15. IF PATIENT HAS HAD SAME OR SIMILAR ILLNESS. GIVE FIRST DATE MM | DD | YY
16. DATES PATIENT UNABLE TO WORK IN CURRENT OCCUPATION FROM MM | DD | YY TO MM | DD | YY
17. NAME OF REFERRING PHYSICIAN OR OTHER SOURCE
17a. I.D. NUMBER OF REFERRING PHYSICIAN
18. HOSPITALIZATION DATES RELATED TO CURRENT SERVICES FROM MM | DD | YY TO MM | DD | YY
19. RESERVED FOR LOCAL USE
20. OUTSIDE LAB? YES NO $ CHARGES
21. DIAGNOSIS OR NATURE OF ILLNESS OR INJURY. (RELATE ITEMS 1,2,3 OR 4 TO ITEM 24E BY LINE)
1. 2. 3. 4.
22. MEDICAID RESUBMISSION CODE ORIGINAL REF. NO.
23. PRIOR AUTHORIZATION NUMBER
24. A B C D E F G H I J K

SPACE 19: RESERVED FOR LOCAL USE: BUYER BEWARE

Although **Space 19** says that it is reserved for local use, there are a host of things that you should place in this spot depending upon the situation. See these below:

a. **Attending Physician, Not Hospice Employee**: Enter the statement "Attending physician, not hospice employee" when a physician renders services to a hospice patient, but the hospice providing the patient's care (in which the patient resides) does not employ the attending physician.

b. **Chiropractic Services**: Enter a six or eight-digit date for the beginning of the services.

c. **Dental Examinations**: Enter the specific surgery for which the exam is being performed.

d. **Foot Care Claims**: Enter a six or eight-digit date the patient was last seen and the NPI of the attending provider when an independent physical or occupational therapist or physician submits the claim.

e. **Homebound Patients**: When an independent lab renders an EKG tracing or obtains a specimen from a homebound or institutionalized patient, enter the word "Homebound" in this space.

f. **Low Osmolar Contrast Material**. Enter the name and dosage amount when low osmolar contrast material is billed, but only if HCPCS codes do not describe them.

g. **Modifier –99**: If you are using the Multiple Modifier (-99) in **Space 24d**, be sure to list the modifiers that the -99 refers to in this space. If you are using the modifier –99 on several lines and on several **CPT** codes in **Space 24d**, be sure to list the multiple modifiers for each line. For example, let's say that you had listed multiple modifiers on a **CPT** code found in the first line on **Space 24d,** as well as on the third line. You would write 1 = (-52,-76); 3 = (-22,-51), indicating that on the first line, the **CPT** was a Reduced Rervice (-52) and a Repeat Procedure (-76), and the code on line three **(Space 24d)** was an Unusual (-22) and Multiple Service (-51).

h. **National Emphysema Treatment Claims**: Enter the number "30" in this space for all national emphysema treatment trial claims.

i. **NOS**: Not Otherwise Classified. If you are submitting a claim for not otherwise classified drugs, enter the drug's name and dosage here.

j. **Patient Refuses to Assign Benefits**: When the beneficiary absolutely refuses to assign benefits to a participating provider, enter "Patient Refuses to Assign Benefits" in this space. In cases such as these, please tell the patient that no payment may be made on the claim.

k. **Shared Postoperative Care**: Enter a six or eight-digit date (either the assumed or relinquished date) for a global surgery when providers share postoperative care.

l. **Testing for Hearing Aid**: Enter the statement "Testing for Hearing Aid" when billing services involving the testing of a hearing aid(s) are used to obtain intentional denials when other payers are involved.

m. **Unlisted Procedure Code**: Enter a concise description of an "unlisted procedure code" or an NOC code if one can be given within the confines of this box. If not, include an attachment with the claim.

Space 20. Outside Lab. This space is to be used if you are billing for diagnostic tests subject to purchase price limitations. If you check the YES box, it will indicate that someone else other than the entity billing for the service (an outside lab) performed the diagnostic service. If you check the YES box, you must also complete **Space 32,** which asks for the name and address of the facility where the services were rendered. If you are billing for multiple-purchased diagnostic tests, each test must be submitted on a separate claim form.

If you check NO in this space, you will have indicated that there were no purchased tests included on this claim form.

The Nitty Gritty

Spaces 21 through 24 are where the money for you is (or is not). **Space 21** (for diagnosis) is where you should indicate the patient's condition or diagnosis. You must use an ICD-9-CM code number. Remember: the higher the number of digits you use for the ICD-9-CM code number (i.e., five digits is better than three because it more fully describes the condition or diagnosis), the better. Diagnoses must be entered in order of priority; that is, list the primary first, the secondary second, and tertiary diagnosis or condition third.

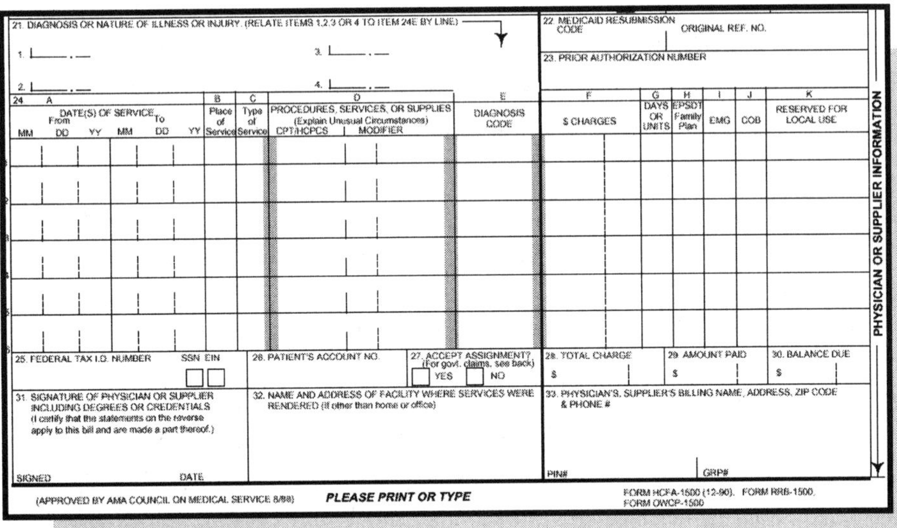

21. DIAGNOSIS OR NATURE OF ILLNESS OR INJURY. (RELATE ITEMS 1,2,3 OR 4 TO ITEM 24E BY LINE)

1. ___ . __   3. ___ . __

2. ___ . __   4. ___ . __

22. MEDICAID RESUBMISSION CODE | ORIGINAL REF. NO.

23. PRIOR AUTHORIZATION NUMBER

24 A						B	C	D		E	F	G	H	I	J	K
DATE(S) OF SERVICE From			To			Place of Service	Type of Service	PROCEDURES, SERVICES, OR SUPPLIES (Explain Unusual Circumstances)		DIAGNOSIS CODE	$ CHARGES	DAYS OR UNITS	EPSDT Family Plan	EMG	COB	RESERVED FOR LOCAL USE
MM	DD	YY	MM	DD	YY			CPT/HCPCS	MODIFIER							

25. FEDERAL TAX I.D. NUMBER SSN EIN

26. PATIENT'S ACCOUNT NO.

27. ACCEPT ASSIGNMENT? (For govt. claims, see back) YES NO

28. TOTAL CHARGE $

29. AMOUNT PAID $

30. BALANCE DUE $

31. SIGNATURE OF PHYSICIAN OR SUPPLIER INCLUDING DEGREES OR CREDENTIALS (I certify that the statements on the reverse apply to this bill and are made a part thereof.)

SIGNED DATE

32. NAME AND ADDRESS OF FACILITY WHERE SERVICES WERE RENDERED (If other than home or office)

33. PHYSICIAN'S, SUPPLIER'S BILLING NAME, ADDRESS, ZIP CODE & PHONE #

PIN# GRP#

PHYSICIAN OR SUPPLIER INFORMATION

(APPROVED BY AMA COUNCIL ON MEDICAL SERVICE 8/88) **PLEASE PRINT OR TYPE** FORM HCFA-1500 (12-90), FORM RRB-1500, FORM OWCP-1500

Listing diagnoses in order of priority is especially important, but there is one exception to this rule. When a new patient comes to your office, make sure that you list the patient's complaint as the primary diagnosis, and then list any and all other diagnoses in order of priority following the complaint.

For example, let's say that a 67-year old female patient came to your office for the first time complaining of blurry vision. If you performed a complete vision screening, completed a history and exam, and decided that the patient had cataracts, you should not list the cataracts as the primary diagnosis. Because the patient was new to your office, you should list the patient's complaint as the primary diagnosis and the cataracts as the secondary diagnosis.

hint

For a Medicare patient NEW to your office, make sure that you list the patient's complaint as the primary diagnosis. If you don't, the claim could be denied.

Space 22, which requests the Medicaid resubmission code, is not required by Medicare and should be left blank.

Space 23 is where you should enter the Professional Review Organization (PRO) prior authorization number for those services requiring PRO prior approval. If an investigational device is used in an FDA-approved clinical trial, you should enter the Investigational Device Exemption number here. For physicians performing care plan oversight services, please enter the 6-digit Medicare provider number of the home health agency (HHA) or hospice when the **CPT** code 99375 or 99376 is used or when the HCPCS National Codes G0064, G0065 or G0066 are billed. Finally, if you are billing for lab services performing CLIA covered procedures, please list the Clinical Laboratory Improvement Act (CLIA) certification number for lab procedures.

Now to the place where you will get paid or not get paid.

Getting Your Claim Paid

Space 24. It is here that you are supposed to gel the information that you have been learning in **CP"Teach"**. Notice that there are dates of service that need to be listed in **Space 24a**. As with other dates needed for the form, make sure that you put either the complete 6 or 8-digit date in this space. Do not worry about listing the dates chronologically as the computer will be able to figure out who did what and when with the dates you supply. What you need to worry about is placing your major service first, followed by the next one, and so on down the line. This will help insure that you receive the best payment possible for the ENTIRE claim. Remember that many claims are paid (although they say this isn't supposed to happen) at a rate equal to 80% of what is listed as the first **CPT** code charge, 50% of the next, and so on down the line. If you are listing things chronologically, chances are the charges for the first few items (e.g., going to the emergency room on a Sunday) will be lower than those for the surgery you may have had to perform. Listing them first may result in your being paid at an 80% on the ER visit and a 50% or 33% rate on the surgery.

If you enter dates that are "to-from," make sure that you list the number of days as "units" (see **Space 24g** for the units or days).

The information requested in **Space 24b** is critical. This tells the insurance company where the service was performed. Back in the old days (before 1990), coders used to write things like "O" if the service occurred in the office. Those days are gone, and it is important to make sure that you use the following table for the place of service codes. These should also be found on the back of an original HCFA 1500 claim form.

11 Office
12 Home
21 Inpatient Hospital
22 Outpatient Hospital
23 Emergency Room –Hospital
24 Ambulatory Surgical Center
25 Birthing Center
26 Military Treatment Facility
31 Skilled Nursing Facility
32 Nursing Facility
33 Custodial Care Facility
34 Hospice
41 Ambulance
42 Ambulance
50 Federally Qualified Health Center
51 Inpatient Psychiatric Facility
52 Psychiatric Facility Partial Hospitalization
53 Community Mental Health Center
54 Intermediate Care Facility/Mentally Retarded
55 Residential Substance Abuse Treatment Facility
56 Psychiatric residential Treatment Center
60 Mass Immunization Center
61 Comprehensive Inpatient Rehabilitation Facility
62 Comprehensive Outpatient Rehabilitation Facility
65 End-Stage Renal Disease
71 State or Local Public Health Clinic
72 Rural Health Clinic

81 Independent Laboratory
99 Other Unlisted Facility

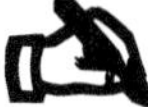

Notice that not all the numbers between 0 and 100 are used. The numbers not being used (e.g., 10) have been unassigned and are available for future use.

Space 24c, which requests the "type" of service, is not required by Medicare.

Space 24d is where you will place the codes of the different procedures that you did. You will need to enter either a **CPT** code or a HCPCS National (Level II) code in this box. Make sure that you do not try to squeeze in any narrative for the description. You will also be able to put in any **CPT** or HCPCS Level II modifier here. Remember, if you have more than two modifiers that apply to one **CPT** code, you will need to use the modifier –99 to indicate to the computer at Medicare's office that you are reporting two or more modifiers. If this is the case, enter the –99 following the **CPT** code (in **Space 24d**) and then enter the different modifiers that apply in **Space 19** as was described above.

If you need to use an unlisted procedure code, place the unlisted procedure code number in the space for 24d, and then in **Space 19**, describe (as concisely as you can) what was done. If the service(s) you performed is/are greater than what you can describe in **Space 19**, be sure to send in a special report. If not, you will only get reimbursed part of what you thought you should get and may have to resubmit your claim.

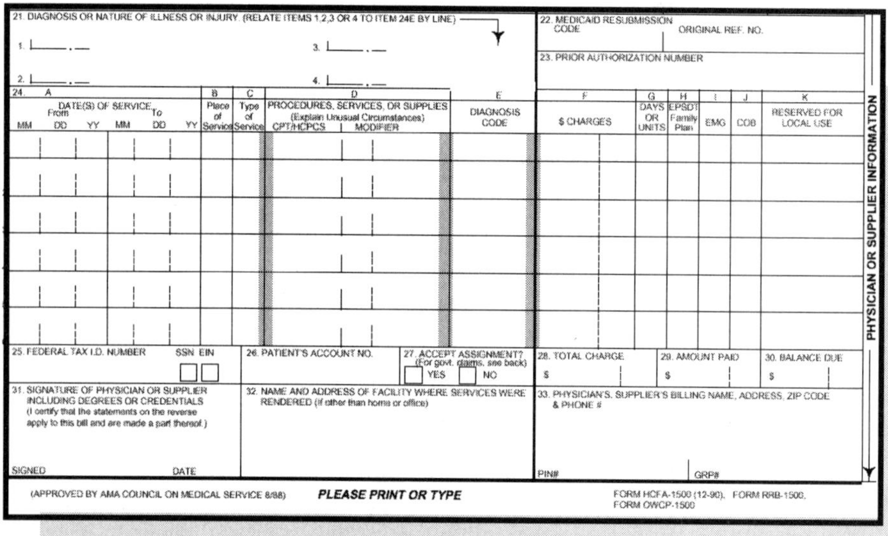

21. DIAGNOSIS OR NATURE OF ILLNESS OR INJURY. (RELATE ITEMS 1,2,3 OR 4 TO ITEM 24E BY LINE)

1. ___ . ___
2. ___ . ___
3. ___ . ___
4. ___ . ___

22. MEDICAID RESUBMISSION CODE | ORIGINAL REF. NO.

23. PRIOR AUTHORIZATION NUMBER

24. A						B	C	D	E	F	G	H	I	J	K
DATE(S) OF SERVICE From			To			Place of Service	Type of Service	PROCEDURES, SERVICES, OR SUPPLIES (Explain Unusual Circumstances) CPT/HCPCS | MODIFIER	DIAGNOSIS CODE	$ CHARGES	DAYS OR UNITS	EPSDT Family Plan	EMG	COB	RESERVED FOR LOCAL USE
MM	DD	YY	MM	DD	YY										

25. FEDERAL TAX I.D. NUMBER SSN EIN

26. PATIENT'S ACCOUNT NO.

27. ACCEPT ASSIGNMENT? (For govt. claims, see back) YES NO

28. TOTAL CHARGE $

29. AMOUNT PAID $

30. BALANCE DUE $

31. SIGNATURE OF PHYSICIAN OR SUPPLIER INCLUDING DEGREES OR CREDENTIALS (I certify that the statements on the reverse apply to this bill and are made a part thereof.)

SIGNED DATE

32. NAME AND ADDRESS OF FACILITY WHERE SERVICES WERE RENDERED (If other than home or office)

33. PHYSICIAN'S, SUPPLIER'S BILLING NAME, ADDRESS, ZIP CODE & PHONE #

PIN# GRP#

PHYSICIAN OR SUPPLIER INFORMATION

(APPROVED BY AMA COUNCIL ON MEDICAL SERVICE 8/88) ***PLEASE PRINT OR TYPE*** FORM HCFA-1500 (12-90), FORM RRB-1500, FORM OWCP-1500

Space 24e is where you relate the diagnosis code to the service you performed. Many people fail to fill out this space, causing lots of rejected claims. Carriers want you to complete **Space 24e** so they can make sure that they are paying you for something that was necessary.

For example, let's say that a patient came in to your office complaining of headaches and rectal bleeding. Let's also say that you "scoped" the patient in the office. If you placed the code for the office visit and the "scope" in **Space 24d** and then only placed the diagnosis code for the headache on the claim form, you may get paid for the office visit and would probably be denied on the scope. This is simply because a "scope" is not the treatment of choice for headaches!

Remember from our discussion of **Space 21** that you should have placed the diagnoses in order from major to minor. This is always true except in cases where the patient is considered to be a "new" patient. In the case of a new patient, you must enter the patient's complaint as the primary diagnosis. Because of this *ordering* from major to minor, you will be able to place the number (i.e., 1,2,3,or 4) in the space marked 24e next to the **CPT** code it goes with.

In the example listed above (the headaches and rectal bleeding), you would have had the ICD-9-CM code for rectal bleeding listed first (next to the number one in **Space 21**) and the code for the headaches listed next (next to the two in **Space 21**). The **CPT** code for the scope would have been listed first with the number "1" placed in **Space 24e,** and the office visit would have been listed second with the numbers "1,2" in **Space 24e**. (For Medicare purposes, in cases where there may be two diagnoses that match a procedure [**CPT** or Level II code(s)]), they prefer that you pick the major diagnosis for that particular service and only list it next to each **CPT** code in **Space 24e**.)

Space 24f requires you to place your charges on the claim form. Once again, place the charges as they correspond to the **CPT** or HCPCS Level II codes (line by line). DO NOT DISCOUNT ANY CHARGES.

hint

Discounting charges in Space 24f on the HCFA 1500 claim form will result in your getting much less for your services than you need. Always charge full fee for everything and let the carriers do the reductions (if any).

If you are charging for hospital visits that occurred over a few days, you will need to make sure that the charge placed in **Space 24f** reflects the total number of days you are charging for. For example, let's say that your patient was in the hospital from January 1st through the 6th. After charging for the initial hospital admission on the first day, you would place the codes (assuming that they were all the same) for the hospital follow-up visits and mark "5" (for five follow-up days) in the units column in **Space 24g**. The charge you would place in **Space 24f** (charge column) would be equal to five times the charge you make for that code for a single day (e.g., if your charge for a single day for the hospital visit is $120, the price you would place in **Space 24f** would be $120 x 5 or $600).

Space 24g, The days or units field, is very important when it comes to telling the carrier how many of a particular ***"like"*** thing you did (e.g., how many "days" in the hospital). This field is most commonly used for multiple visits, units of supplies, anesthesia minutes [always list the total number of minutes (not hours) for total anesthesia time or oxygen volume]. This field must be completed, even if only one unit was provided (e.g., even if you did the surgery once or the patient had one day in the hospital).

Spaces 24h and i (EPSDT/EMG) are not required by Medicare and should be left blank.

Spaces 24j and k are for "COB" and "reserved for local use." Medicare requests that you use these spaces to enter in the NPI (National Provider Identifier) of the person providing the services if they are part of a group practice. The way that you will do this is to enter the first two digits of the NPI in **Space 24j** and then the balance (the remaining six digits) of the number in **Space 24k** including the two-digit location identifier.

Space 25 (Federal Tax I.D.) is where you will place the provider of service or supplier Federal Tax I.D. number or Social Security Number. This number is required for any Medigap transfer of information.

Space 26 is where you will place the patient's account number that you have in your office (i.e., the number that helps you keep your records straight). It will help you in your patient's identification. Medicare will return any of the account numbers listed here to you.

ACCEPTING ASSIGNMENT

In **Space 27**, you will need to indicate whether or not you will accept assignment for this claim. Accepting assignment means that you agree that you will accept payment from Medicare as the payment in full (for all covered services) on the patient's behalf (after he has met his deductible, of course, and has paid the co-pay). That is, you will not bill the patient for any additional monies on covered services after Medicare has made its payment to you.

Remember, if there is a Medigap policy and if you have indicated this in **Space 9** and have gotten the authorization from the patient and/or authorized representative to receive Medigap benefits, you will need to be a "participating" provider or supplier, and you must accept assignment of Medicare benefits for all covered charges for the patient.

There are six types of providers of service or suppliers and claims that can be paid on an "assignment" basis. These include:

a. Clinical diagnostic laboratory services

b. Physician services to patients entitled to both Medicare and Medicaid

c. "Participating" physician or supplier services

d. Ambulatory Surgical Center services for covered Ambulatory Surgical Center (ASC) procedures

e. Home dialysis supplies and equipment paid under Method II (see **Medicare Supplier Manual** for more information on Method II)

f. Services of the following persons:

   1. physician's assistants;
   2. nurse practitioners;
   3. clinical nurse specialists;

4. nurse midwives;
5. certified registered anesthetists;
6. clinical psychologists;
7. clinical social workers.

Space 28 requires that you total all of the charges for your services (total of **Space 24f**) and place that number in this box.

Space 29 will be where you place the amount of money that the patient has paid for ***covered services only***. Do not place the total amount the patient has paid for all of the services if all of them are not covered by Medicare. For example, let's say that your patient came in for an ophthalmological visit, and let's say that you performed an intermediate established-patient visit for ophthalmology (see code 92012). Let's say that you also determined the refractive state (see code 92105). This code, 92015, is not covered by Medicare. Therefore, if the patient paid you her 20% co-pay for the office visit and all of the money for the determination of the refractive state, you would only report the 20% that the patient paid you for the office visit in **Space 29**. The reason for this is that the 20% for the office visit is the only service that you provided that was "covered" by Medicare.

Even though **Space 30** asks you for the total amount due by the patient, this is not required by Medicare, and you can just leave it blank.

In **Space 31** (Signature of Physician or Supplier), have the physician sign the form, indicating that he or she has seen it and that the services outlined there were in fact provided. You will also need to enter either the 6 or

8-digit date here (or the alpha-numeric alternative), indicating the date that the form was signed. Even though Medicare allows an authorized representative to sign in this box, remember that this only increases the chances for you (if you are the "authorized representative") being just as liable (if things go wrong) as the person you are coding for. Also, there are instances in some offices where people will falsify claims only to get the money for themselves and use the office "stamp" as your signature (if you are the doctor). This only adds to the problems of fraud and abuse.

Space 32 calls for the name and address of the facility if the services were furnished in a hospital, clinic, laboratory, or facility other than the patient's home or physician's office. When the name and address of the facility where the services were provided is the same as the name and address shown in **Space 33**, enter the word "Same".

Last but not least, **Space 33** calls for the provider of service/supplier's billing name, address, zip code, and telephone number. Enter the National Provider Identifier (NPI) (including the two-digit identifier) for the performing provider of service/supplier who either IS or is NOT a member of a group practice.

By following the steps to fill out the HCFA 1500 claim form correctly, and by properly coding both your ICD-9-CM and **CPT** codes, you will experience fewer rejections of claims, increased processing efficiency, and higher/more accurate reimbursements. Your patients will also appreciate the fact that they will owe lower balances, as the insurance carrier will have paid correctly. Good Luck!

Summary

CHAPTER TWELVE

- ✔ Always complete the HCFA 1500 claim form following the directions outlined on the form.

- ✔ Remember that there are some spaces on the form that are not filled in (for Medicare) exactly according to what is asked for on the claim form. Examples include Space 24 j and k.

- ✔ Failure to complete the HCFA 1500 properly could result in failure by the carrier to pay the claim.

- ✔ Remember that failure to relate the diagnosis code to the **CPT** code will result in a denial of the claim.

- ✔ Always list the **CPT** codes from major to minor. Do not list the codes chronologically (according to what happened first, second, third and so on), unless you are coding for a new patient, in which case you must list the initial reasons for the visit first.

- ✔ Remember to list your diagnosis codes from the primary diagnosis code on down.

- ✔ In the case of a new Medicare patient, be sure to list the patient's complaint as the primary diagnosis.

Index

A

Adjunct codes 378
Alpha-numeric 18
AMA CPT-4 Advisory Committee 41
American Dental Association 44
Anatomic and Surgical Pathology 332
Anatomical order 308
Anesthesia, by surgeon 413
Anesthesia code 15
Anesthesia Section 44
Appendix A, CPT 401
Application of Casts and Strapping 258

B

Bullet 312

C

Cardiovascular System 196
Chemistry and Toxicology 331
Code usage 188
Completing Your HCFA 1500 Claim Form for Medicare 449
Complex repair 249, 253, 416
CPT Surgical Package 204
Critical Care Services 162-164
Current Procedural Terminology 52
Custodial Services 174

D

Detailed History 95-96
Diagnostic Procedures 205
DOC form 118-123
Doctor's Office Checklist 118

E

Established patient 84
Evaluation and Management Section 83–90, 405
Examinations 100–101
Expanded Problem Focused History 93–94

F

Face-To-Face Prolonged Services 176
Female genital system 283
Five-digit numeric codes 39
Follow-up Inpatient Consultation 154–155
Foreign body 223, 225, 227

G

Gross examination 341
Guidelines 46, 196, 209, 242, 309, 327

H

Handling code 380
Health Care Financing Administration 7, 20
Home Services 176

I

Indefinite post-ops 225
Indefinite pre-ops 225
Initial cast placement 255
Initial Hospital Care 141
Injectable substances, coding for 356
Intermediate repair 246
Invasive 377
Invasive procedures 377
Inverted triangles 312, 351

K

Key component 87

L

Logic of National Codes 18

M

Major to minor 258
Maternity Care 286, 289
Medicare 375
Medicare Follow-up Care 208
Medicare policy, follow-up care 207
Medicare program 7
Medicare Surgical Package 201
Medicine Section 17, 351–365
Miscellaneous Codes 332
Modifier -22 281, 310, 330, 400
Modifier -51 251, 253
Modifier -52 402
Modifier -62 (two surgeons) 423
Modifier -75 148
Modifier -76 256
Modifier -77 256
Modifier -99 404, 421, 432
Modifiers 400
Multiple Procedures 212
Musculoskeletal System 195

N

"N/C" charge 381
NATIONAL 20
National Coding Manual 9, 44, 357
New patient 84
Noninvasive 17
Noninvasive procedures 376, 377
Noninvasive services 197
Notes 242
Numbering System (CPT) 43
Numeric digits 13

O

OBRA law 20
Omnibus Budget Reconciliation Act 86, 258

P

Pathology and Laboratory Section 16, 44, 327–329

Physician travels 389
Physician's supervision 327
Placement of casts and strapping 255
Post-op 204
Postoperative care 240
Problem Focused History 92
Prolonged Services 176

R

Radiology Section 16, 44
Reduced services 419
Repair, types of 246
Respiratory System 196
Rest Home 174

S

Simple repair 247
Special report 232, 309, 330, 331, 406
Starred procedures 379
Subsequent Hospital Care 141
Supervision and interpretation 311
Supplies and materials 237, 386
Surgery 204
Surgery Section 15, 44, 196, 228, 232, 377
Surgical Package 199, 223, 420
Surgical Pathology 335

T

Telephone calls 180–181
Therapeutic or diagnostic injections 355
Time 405
Triangle 312
Two surgeons 425

U

Unlisted procedure 218, 309, 329
Unusual circumstances 330
Unusual service 400

V

Visit codes 85